INTERDISCIPLINARY RESEARCH

INTERDISCIPLINARY RESEARCH
Diverse Approaches in Science, Technology, Health and Society

Edited by
PROFESSOR JOHN ATKINSON
University of Paisley
PROFESSOR MALCOLM CROWE
University of Paisley

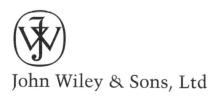

John Wiley & Sons, Ltd

Copyright © 2006   John Wiley & Sons Ltd
             The Atrium, Southern Gate, Chichester,
             West Sussex PO19 8SQ, England
             Telephone (+44) 1243 779777

Email (for orders and customer service enquiries): cs-books@wiley.co.uk
Visit our Home Page on www.wiley.com

Other Wiley Editorial Offices

John Wiley & Sons Inc., 111 River Street, Hoboken, NJ 07030, USA

Jossey-Bass, 989 Market Street, San Francisco, CA 94103-1741, USA

Wiley-VCH Verlag GmbH, Boschstr. 12, D-69469 Weinheim, Germany

John Wiley & Sons Australia Ltd, 42 McDougall Street, Milton, Queensland 4064, Australia

John Wiley & Sons (Asia) Pte Ltd, 2 Clementi Loop #02-01, Jin Xing Distripark, Singapore 129809

John Wiley & Sons Canada Ltd, 6045 Freemont Blvd, Mississauga, ONT L5R

Wiley also publishes its books in a variety of electronic formats. Some content that appears in print may not be available in electronic books.

Library of Congress Cataloging-in-Publication Data
Interdisciplinary research : diverse approaches in science, technology,
     health, and society / edited by John Atkinson and Malcolm Crowe.
          p. ; cm.
     Includes bibliographical references and index.
     ISBN-13: 978-1-86156-470-2 (paper : alk. paper)
     ISBN-10: 1-86156-470-8 (paper : alk. paper)
     1. Social medicine–Miscellanea.   2. Technology–Miscellanea.
3. Health–Miscellanea.   4. Science–Miscellanea.   I. Atkinson, John,
PhD.   II. Crowe, M. K. (Malcolm K.)
     [DNLM: 1. Ethics, Research.   2. Research–methods.   3. Interdisci-
plinary Communication.   W 20.5 I5145 2006]
     RA418.I58 2006
     362.1–dc22
                                                        2006011235

A catalogue record for this book is available from the British Library
ISBN-13 978-1-86156-470-2
ISBN-10 1-86156-470-8

Typeset by SNP Best-set Typesetter Ltd., Hong Kong
Printed and bound in Great Britain by TJ International Ltd, Padstow, Cornwall

This book is printed on acid-free paper responsibly manufactured from sustainable forestry in which at least two trees are planted for each one used for paper production.

Contents

Contributors

Professor John Atkinson is Professor and Associate Dean in the School of Health Nursing and Midwifery at the University of Paisley. He comes from a community nursing background with clinical, management and academic experience particularly with marginalised people. Before entering universities he was health care manager at HM Prison Barlinnie. Among his publications are: *Nursing Homeless Men* (2000), chapters on HIV/AIDS and homelessness, and research-based articles.

Professor Malcolm Crowe gained his DPhil in Mathematics from Oxford in 1979, becoming Head of Computing in Paisley in 1985, where he introduced an 'interpretivist' degree in Information Systems. From the resulting culture clash, university-level research development, and hundreds of Masters students, he has gained a multidisciplinary view of research.

Professor Neil Blain is Professor of Media and Culture in the School of Media, Language and Music at the University of Paisley. Recent books include the co-authored *Media, Monarchy and Power*, and *Sport, Media, Culture: Local and Global Dimensions* (both 2003). He co-edits *The International Journal of Media and Cultural Politics*.

Professor Ian Boyd is Professor of Biology and Director of the NERC Sea Mammal Research Unit at the University of St Andrews. He is a Fellow of the Royal Society of Edinburgh and a recipient of the Bruce Medal for polar science, the Scientific Medal of the Zoological Society of London and the Marshall Award for Freshwater and Marine Conservation. He is an editor of the *Journal of Zoology* and an honorary professor at the University of Birmingham. Until 2001, he was a programme principal investigator for the British Antarctic Survey.

Mr Mario Hair has been a statistics lecturer at the University of Paisley for the last eighteen years. He is also active within the Statistics Consultancy Unit based at the university. His research interests include survey methodology. As a consultant he has completed projects for a wide range of clients.

Professor Andrew S. Hursthouse is a Professor in the School of Engineering and Science, University of Paisley. He is an environmental geochemist and Chartered Chemist, with research interests developing from an 'Earth systems' approach to applied and industrial issues, supporting sustainable development. He collaborates with researchers nationally and internationally on waste and pollution management issues and has a strong interest in environmental regulation and policy development.

Professor John MacDonald is Professor of Psychology in the School of Social Sciences at the University of Paisley. He is a Chartered Psychologist and an Associate Fellow of the British Psychological Society. His most well-known research is in the area of auditory-visual speech processing, where he was one of the discoverers of the 'McGurk' effect.

Dr Harriet Mowat is the Managing Director of Mowat Research Ltd, a research and development company which focuses on the ageing population and the practical implications for social change. She is a senior research associate of the University of Paisley School of Nursing and Midwifery. Her research interests include spirituality and ageing, successful ageing in the workplace and collaboration.

Professor Martin Myant is a Professor in Paisley Business School at the University of Paisley. He has written on economic and political development in east-central Europe. His latest book, *The Rise and Fall of Czech Capitalism: Economic Development in the Czech Republic since 1989*, was published by Edward Elgar in 2003.

Professor Nigel Rapport is a social anthropologist. He holds the Canada Research Chair in Globalization, Citizenship and Justice at Concordia University of Montreal, where he is Founding Director of the Centre for Cosmopolitan Studies. He is also Professor at the Norwegian University of Science and Technology, Trondheim. He has been elected a Fellow of the Royal Society of Edinburgh. His research interests include social theory, phenomenology, identity and individuality, community, conversation analysis, and links between anthropology and literature and philosophy.

Professor P. Anne Scott was appointed Deputy President of Dublin City University in February 2006. She has worked clinically and as an academic in Ireland, Scotland and Kenya. Anne's research interests are in the philosophy and ethics of health care and in judgement and decision-making on issues of ethics and clinical practice.

Professor John Swinton holds the chair in Practical Theology and Pastoral Care at the University of Aberdeen. He worked for 16 years as a registered nurse specialising in psychiatry and learning disabilities. He also worked for a number of years as a community mental health chaplain. In 2004 he founded the Centre for Spirituality, Health and Disability at the University of

Aberdeen, a research centre with a dual focus on the relationship between spirituality and health and the theology of disability.

Dr Abel Usoro lectures in the School of Computing, University of Paisley, Scotland. His research interests are information systems and knowledge management for which he has been widely published in refereed international conferences, journals and book chapters. He is a member of both the Information Institute and the British Computing Society.

Preface

This book is for research activists, especially those involved in education institutions and research degrees. Its journey started at the University of Paisley with the establishment of a Post Graduate Certificate in Research Degree Supervision. A number of colleagues from a variety of disciplines came together to promote research activity and help colleagues undertake supervision.

At first it appeared simple enough, as each discipline from the 'hard' or 'soft' area of research endeavour presented its perspective. The discussion, however, was less clear and much more exciting. Assumptions and long-held beliefs brought to the gatherings were certainly challenged, influenced and sometimes profoundly changed. The working title for this book was 'a celebration of research approaches' to reflect this vibrant interaction. From these activities the editors approached the authors in this book to portray their perspectives and enrich the debate.

One overriding theme, presented in this book, is how all parties tend to recognise multiple approaches to answering questions. This has been a surprise to some of our more qualitatively based colleagues, who tended to consider empirical scientists as only 'believing' their own research. Conversely, quantitatively weighted individuals have become familiar with the need for qualitative approaches, in particular, of how 'bilingual' approaches often enrich research studies, providing depth and practical insight into how the 'science' can be transferred to humanity. This is particularly important in research related to the provision of public service and the spending of public money.

Another theme was the need, in all approaches, for rigour and clarity, to establish the questions and choose the methodology that would address them, not necessarily just those to which one is accustomed. Alongside this was the search and development of the 'likely story' and how important this is to all research disciplines. This book does not pretend to be comprehensive in terms of including all kinds of research. It does, it is hoped, convey approaches from perspectives right across the continuum of research.

Similarly, the book does not purport to tell the reader how to carry out collaborative, multidisciplinary research. Rather its purpose is to provide windows into a variety of approaches. It is hoped that, armed with this information and insight, readers will consider their research questions and challenges from a broader base. This may be seen as good academic practice, but the authors also hope that practical benefits may accrue as well – funding bodies have put an increased emphasis on multidisciplinary, collaborative research.

Finally, we sincerely hope that the reader will enjoy the book and gain a feeling of the fun that debate and pursuing research engenders in us all.

John Atkinson and Malcolm Crowe
University of Paisley, January 2006

1 Research Today

MALCOLM CROWE

School of Computing, University of Paisley, UK

INTRODUCTION

This book contains research papers taken from a dozen or so different disciplines. It is striking that they nearly all seem to share a common view of what research is, how it should be carried on, and of course, how it should be written up. Moreover, these common features can be traced back four hundred years, to Francis Bacon (1620), and before. It is equally striking, however, that these common features seem to have been quite rarely discussed in recent times, so that this chapter can perhaps claim to be a rediscovery of age-old research methods. It is offered in homage to all researchers who have discovered these paths for themselves, and as a gift to all who have not.

Some writings on research would lead us to expect that research, at least within scientific subjects, would exhibit the 'scientific method', by which many people seem to mean the hypothetico-deductive method (Whewell 1837). Others might lead us to expect methods advocated for qualitative research, such as grounded theory (Glaser & Strauss 1967). Some writers on how research should be conducted try to impose epistemological rules (empiricism, positivism and the like). While examples of all of these things may be found in doctoral theses, few academic journals appear to contain examples of such methods, even in their home disciplines. There are only two primary quantitative research papers in the collection, and only one of them, on marine biology, uses the hypothetico-deductive approach, and then only to make tentative suggestions for an algorithm.

Instead, the most striking recurring aspect in the research papers presented here is that the reader often seems to be invited to accompany the researcher on a journey of discovery. The invitation is of course rarely explicit, but often the research paper can be read as an account of a sort of journey that points out things found on the way, notes what others have found on similar travels, and gives a tentative explanation of what has been discovered. On such a reading we might imagine that the researcher hopes that the readers will find similar things for themselves on future journeys, and to this extent the researcher seems to infer paradigms of what to look for. It is only rarely that

Interdisciplinary Research: Diverse Approaches in Science, Technology, Health and Society.
Edited by J. Atkinson and M. Crowe.
Copyright © 2006 by John Wiley & Sons, Ltd.

the author goes beyond such stereotypes to suggest a theoretical basis for what has been seen, and rarer still for the author to make any claims that a natural law has been discovered.

Another aspect that seems to be common across the exemplars is an academic, scholarly style. This aims for an impersonal stance and a wide audience, including, but not limited to, an academic community studying questions similar to those considered in the research paper. Since the knowledge is new, it is to be expected that some readers will be surprised by the result, and may feel disposed to disagree. The style is therefore chosen to be careful and cogent in leading the reader to its conclusions, cautious in its interpretation, and to avoid any writing that invites dismissal because it looks like opinion, hearsay or prejudice.

Thirdly, there seems to be a widely shared confidence as to what counts as evidence worth placing before the reader. Offering such evidence is not the same as making a truth claim, or claiming any privileged standpoint, such as objectivity. As noted above, instead of magisterial assertions of objective fact, we find in these papers that the readers are merely invited to consider the evidence for themselves.

So far, we have three ingredients: the journey of discovery, the academic style, and the nature of the evidence. It is natural to ask whether these three aspects could possibly be sufficient characteristics of research. That is, will any piece of writing that has these aspects qualify as research? The answer to such a question would turn on what was to be understood by 'discovery', 'academic' or 'evidence'. In these papers, evidence is of course carefully and sparingly selected. For example, the anthropologist's tale has many particularities of the interview subject, but all of the things we are told are of interest to anthropologists – how Bob socialises, eats, lives, relaxes – very much in the style of Margaret Mead (1928). Writers on more trivial matters might be more interested in, say, the number of rooms in Bob's house, the décor, or how to cook his favourite dish.

Thus, naturally, what is being written depends on the discipline, as will the nature of the journey and what counts as an explanation. What counts as retracing the journey will also vary from one discipline to another: is it enough to follow the argument, retracing the journey in the imagination, or is it actually necessary, or feasible, to carry out the steps oneself?

It appears to be widely accepted that the goal of research is new knowledge. From the above discussion we might infer that the templates or stereotypes that have been offered during the journey of discovery may count as new knowledge once the range of applicability of these templates has been established to the satisfaction of the academic community involved. This notion of solidarity, and the attachment to norms of argument, it has been argued (Rorty 1982a), is what we find today in place of the appeals to truth that characterised a previous generation.[1]

---

[1] 'The accident of which glimpses of the world our sense organs have vouchsafed us, and the further accidents of the predicates we have entrenched or the theories whose proportions please us, may determine what we have a right to believe. But how could they determine the *truth*?' (Rorty 1982c, p. 12).

Thus to the three aspects noted above we must add a fourth: the notion of an academic community. This depends on the discipline, and arguably each of our example papers addresses a different community of academics. A good research paper, it seems, is one that deploys the above methods in considering a question of interest to such an academic community – a 'research question'.

Just possibly these four aspects now are sufficient to separate academic research papers from other forms of writing. Popular articles on travel or cookery involve the reader in discovery, and have a definite view of what sorts of information to offer their readers, but possibly lack the academic community; science fiction would have the community, and the shared journey of the imagination, perhaps even discovery in exploration of imagined scenarios (thought-experiments?), but their fictions could hardly count as evidence.

This book intended to be a contribution to a sort of ethnography of research. The plan was to observe what a sample of researchers currently (said they) do, inferring what they value, and postulating a shared enterprise. This opening chapter itself therefore naturally exemplifies the four aspects described above. Thus, in this chapter I hope to lead you to discover these aspects in the papers presented, and, once I have set them out in order, I hope to persuade you that other examples of research that you may encounter will also have these features. And as to the academic community: here it is the rather wide community of all academics, for whom research itself is a natural area of concern.

It must be admitted, however, that, over the collection period, the rather simple methodology of this plan has been damaged by several contributors adding some self-reflective ('philosophical') sections, influenced by drafts of this chapter and outlines of the book as a whole. We have accepted these changes in the belief that your experience as a reader will be the more interesting: you are seeing a snapshot of precisely the sort of cyclical process that characterises our tradition, where every discussion leaves opportunities for further research.

THE JOURNEY OF DISCOVERY

ORIGINS

The modern notion of research dates from the seventeenth century, with Francis Bacon (1561–1626):

> There was but one course left, therefore, – to try the whole thing anew upon a better plan, and to commence a total reconstruction of sciences, arts, and all human knowledge, raised upon the proper foundations. And this, though in the project and undertaking it may seem a thing infinite and beyond the powers of man, yet when it comes to be dealt with it will be found sound and sober, more so than what has been done hitherto. For of this there is some issue; whereas in what is

now done in the matter of science there is only a whirling round about, and perpetual agitation, ending where it began, and although he was well aware how solitary an enterprise it is, and how hard a thing to win faith and credit for, nevertheless he was resolved not to abandon either it or himself; nor to be deterred from trying and entering upon that one path which is alone open to the human mind. For better it is to make a beginning of that which may lead to something, than to engage in a perpetual struggle and pursuit in courses which have no exit. and certainly the two ways of contemplation are much like those two ways of action, so much celebrated, in this – that the one, arduous and difficult in the beginning, leads out at last into the open country; while the other, seeming at first sight easy and free from obstruction, leads to pathless and precipitous places. (Bacon 2000, *Proœmium*)

Here in his description of his project as 'a total reconstruction of sciences, arts and all human knowledge', we see the full breadth of his project, ranging in *The Advancement of Learning* (1605) from Natural Philosophy in Book 1 to Human Philosophy in Book 2, including that of the individual and of society (civil). We also see the analogy of the 'one path which is alone open to the human mind', the journey of discovery, which he uses often in his works (see Figure 1.1). As Lord Chancellor of England, his voice was influential: though he died in 1626, the Royal Society was founded in 1660, and the Académie des Sciences in 1666, and similar bodies followed in other countries. These key institutions themselves form part of a trend towards the development of learned societies, in which the founding of the Académie Française in 1635 is notable. In the seventeenth century science was still closely coupled with magic and alchemy, so that the birth of the scientific tradition was characterised by a careful disavowal of esoteric revelation on the one hand, and popular and ill-informed notions on the other.

(Curiously, the inclusion of science in the university curriculum is due to another Bacon. Roger Bacon's (1214–1294) own contribution was the application of geometry to optics, and an encyclopaedia of science. He knew for example that the earth was round, and that the stars were more than 100 million miles away.)

Francis Bacon's is the first writing in which we see the need set out for the corpus of what we would now call academic knowledge – careful, scholarly, painstaking, precise, fit to be cited in contexts not imagined when it was set down. In the area of natural philosophy such knowledge should be based on direct observation of nature, not hearsay or presumption; and in areas of human philosophy based on careful, intellectual, processes not tied to a foregone conclusion. For four hundred years we have been pursuing this ideal of research, and Bacon would be proud and delighted to see the works that have resulted!

On the other hand, Bacon himself fell into the ancient and common error of imagining that there might be a universal scientific method. He derided Empiricalism, but had overambitious hopes for a new sort of induction that

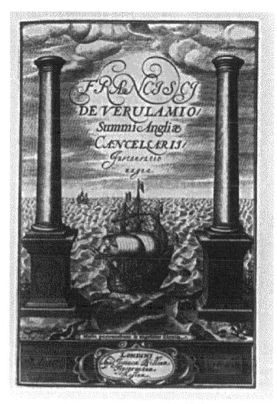

Figure 1.1. The frontispiece of Francis Bacon's *Instauratio Magna* (1620) shows ships sailing beyond the Pillars of Hercules, the classical edge of the known world. The inscription 'Multi pertransibunt et augebitur scientia', famously used in many school mottoes, is presumably from Daniel 12:4, but misquotes the Vulgate and rather poorly translates the Hebrew. (*Source*: Courtesy of Glasgow University Library.)

he set out in Book 2 of *Novum Organum*. Various philosophers have had a go at this problem, from Aristotle to John Stuart Mill. William Whewell, inventor of the word 'scientist', inspired countless PhD theses with his hypothetico-deductive method (1837). In the end, however, all scientists must content themselves with Bacon's endless cycle of moving from observation to hypotheses and back again: this simple notion is in the end what has brought about so much scientific progress. Bacon envisaged knowledge as a hierarchy of 'axioms', building on each other, each painstakingly established through a series of cyclical researches, which people now call inductive generalisation.

Such cycles are not confined to the sciences. There is an endless cycle from individual observations to postulated generalisations in qualitative research. In developing protestant theology, Chladenius devised the hermeneutic circle,

'Complete knowledge always involves an apparent circle, that each part can be understood only out of the whole to which it belongs, and vice versa' (1742, pp. 84–85). The hermeneutic circle was taken up by Schleiermacher, Dilthey (as one of his aporia – problems without solutions), Gadamer, and others in the human sciences.[2]

FELLOW TRAVELLERS

In this book we have a number of exemplars: we can discern the operation of such an agenda in these disparate subject areas.

For example, the environmental geochemist's tale is one of the most 'scientific' articles in this book, but does not follow the hypothetico-deductive 'scientific' paradigm. Instead it uses starkly scientific language to describe some acts of exploration, in which biologists dig up samples in the Clyde estuary, stew them and grind them in careful ways, and come to considered conclusions. But we can detect the cyclical scientific study here rather than the strictly hypothetico-deductive one. The intended audience consists of environmentalists who know in general terms what they are looking for (pollution, sickly life forms), they have established methods for their search, but they are not testing hypotheses. Instead, they are adding to an existing corpus of such findings, and reporting their own findings, so that other researchers can look for similar results in other estuaries or at other times. Their conclusions are not theories, but might allow models to be built at some later time.

The mediarist's tale explicitly looks to alternatives to the scientific, and yet we find very much the same scientific approach. Following a brief review of well-known literary meta-narratives such as 'structuralism', we are led into the writer's world: media and cultural studies research, whose examples, both in the general and more personal sections, are described in quite scientific terms. An account is given of an exploration into the written word and television reportage, on the subject of monarchy: 'this book's main empirical evidence is media content'. The mediarist seems to be thrown by the rejoinder 'what does that prove?' and appears briefly tempted to retreat into ' "true" quantitative work', but the proposal of Bacon's method is that the reader is invited, fol-

---

[2] But the basic dilemma is ancient. Heraclitus (c. 500 BC; Crowe 1996):

συλλαψιες
ολα καιουκ ολα
συμφερομενον διαφερομενον
συναδον διαδον
εκ παντων εν
και εξ ενος παντα

[Concepts: wholes and not wholes, convergent divergent, consonant dissonant, from all things a unity and from this unity all things.]; or Plato's *Meno* (79c), where Socrates asks 'α'λλ' οι'' ει τινὰ ει'δέναι μόριον α'ρετῆς ο'' τι ε'στίν, αυ'τὴν μὴ ει'δότα; [Does anyone know what a part of virtue is, without knowing the whole?]'

lowing this journey and armed with its new insights, to find similar things when we construct a sample ourselves. Above all, we note Bacon's cycle between observation and hypothesis: the researcher has gained impressions from previous output for which he now feels able to provide the evidence by analysis of the words themselves.

Across all disciplines, though, the emphasis is on public (non-esoteric) knowledge: things that can be shown, and possibly explained, to any reader who takes the trouble to follow the progress of the research.

Table 1.1 indicates how the reader of each of our research papers is invited to share a journey of discovery with the author.

Table 1.1. Sharing a journey of discovery

Paper	The invitation to the journey
Environmental geochemist (Chapter 3)	Motivation: dealing with pollution, especially chromium. Softening up: account of sample collection. Leads into: account of processing, and conclusions. Rewards: data on mobility of chromium pollutant.
Mediarist (Chapter 8)	Motivation: study of mass media. Softening up: a promise to discuss academic disciplines. Rewards: a promised critique of contemporary, social and cultural practices.
Spiritual researcher (Chapter 11)	Motivation: widening awareness of spiritual issues in health and social care. Softening up: contrast with the age of individualism versus pursuit of meaning. Leads into: discussion of policy initiatives with this dimension. Rewards: refocusing ideas of health and sickness, and the notion of successful ageing.
Psychologist (Chapter 6)	Motivation: processes involved in speech perception. Softening up: simple ideas of perception and illusion. Leads into: account of experimental studies and theories. Rewards: greater understanding of complexity of processes involved.
Anthropologist (Chapter 9)	Motivation: postmodern approaches to anthropology. Softening up: focus on Bob, the bodybuilder and hospital porter. Leads into: consideration of some wide issues such as 'governmentality' and 'elsewhere'. Rewards: notes towards the perfect biography.
Marine biologist (Chapter 2)	Motivation: continuing debate about impact of predators on fisheries and global warming. Softening up: at its simplest level, just multiply daily ration by population size. Leads into: detailed algorithms and statistics. Rewards: an opportunity to examine overall consumption of prey by marine predators.

Table 1.1. *Continued*

Paper	The invitation to the journey
Information technologist (Chapter 5)	Motivation: how to globalise business operations and markets. Softening up: consider organisation, ICT, personnel, infrastructure. Leads into: survey of interest to strategic managers. Rewards: what is valued, what seems to be missing, what can be done next.
Health policy researcher (Chapter 12)	Motivation: how to improve health care from patient's viewpoint. Softening up: the viewpoint of a rural cancer patient. Leads into: discovery of common themes in stories. Rewards: improvements in health policy.
Nurse philosopher (Chapter 10)	Motivation: contrast the (philosophical) basis of health care research with the 'philosophy' (objectives?) of nursing. Softening up: need for clarity and honesty in addressing evidence. Rewards: evidence-based practice is bound to be better than any dogma.
Statistician (Chapter 4)	Motivation: the plight of the statistician faced with bad experiments. Softening up: anecdotes on wasted research effort. Rewards: thinking about statistics first improves research.
Political historian (Chapter 7)	Motivation: contextualisation of historical evidence. Softening up: different views of Communism in 1978 and now, and the riveting Prague Spring story. Rewards: a new view of history as a reflection of the present.
Chapter 1	Motivation: what is research? Softening up: no heavy theory here, look at what researchers do. Leads into: historical analysis. Rewards: insights into how research papers are written.

OBJECTIVITY AND CONTEXT

We consider now the second ingredient that may be seen as common to all of the contributions: the academic style of the contribution. The author is self-effacing: the narratives presented in research papers are written in an 'impersonal' style. The reader is assumed to have some knowledge of the context. This divorce from the identity of the author and any knowledge of the reader is fundamental to the academic style. In another age we might have called the resulting style objective. It is striking that the author claims no unique qualities or insights: there is the implication that the conclusions being drawn or the procedures being followed are within everyone's capacity; at least everyone with a similar knowledge of the background or prior art.

Researchers who use grammar checkers will notice repeated objections to their use of the passive voice. As in storytelling, the author should not seem to have too many personal characteristics that might get in the way of the story: we should focus on the story and not be distracted by the personality of the author. It is curious that in the twenty-first century, while storytelling continues as before, literary criticism has turned this habit on its head. It seems the public really wants to know everything about Philip Larkin, Kingsley Amis etc. even though it may turn out that biographies, however detailed, shed little light on the literary output of their subjects. Even knowing that a character in a novel is based partly on a real person is scant help in analysis of that character, since the author's view of that person is not necessarily completely reflected in the invented character.

The reader knows some of the context, or they won't read the paper; not all of the context, or the paper is redundant. As a general rule in research papers, the reader is assumed to be a peer in the research discipline, but one who needs to be told about the circumstances of the particular research described in the paper. A paper written for an international conference should take pains to avoid or explain any references to matters that are of local knowledge.

In this section we consider what sort of writing would be acceptable in an academic paper. Many aspects in the above description rely on collective notions of what counts as a consistent account, a valid explanation, a cogent theory etc.

LIKELY STORIES

The phrase 'likely stories' is first recorded in its Greek form, in Plato's *Timaeus* (29):

> Do not therefore be surprised, Socrates, if on many matters concerning the gods and the whole world of change we are unable in every respect and on every occasion to render consistent and accurate account. You must be satisfied if our account is as likely as any, remembering that both I and you who are sitting in judgement on it are merely human, and should not look for anything more than a likely story in such matters.

Plato and later commentators have been dissatisfied with this approach. It has often seemed to lead to the use of many incompatible likely stories: Copernicus complained that:

> With them it is as though an artist were to gather the hands, feet, head and other members for his images from diverse models, each part excellently drawn, but not related to a single body, and since they in no way match each other, the result would be a monster rather than a man. (Kuhn 1992, *The Copernican Revolution*, p. 138)

Following Descartes, common practice has been to allow such stories to convince if they fit together with others to explain many phenomena. Then they become *theories*, and as evidence is gathered, they are refined to become ever more effective. The twin goals are simplicity (or generality – a theory with as few special cases as possible) and efficacy (a theory that, ideally, is sufficient to explain many things).

Many people (Francis Bacon, Ramon Lull, René Descartes, Francis Bacon, Isaac Newton, John Locke, John Stuart Mill, William Whewell, Gottlob Frege, Bertrand Russell, to name but a few) have dreamed that this process could be mechanised, so that with the help of some careful methods and cleverly designed experiments we could make steady progress in decoding the universe, and resolving all its parts. Writers in other branches of research at first rather nervously tried to copy the 'scientific method' or create similarly empiricist alternatives for the social sciences (Burrell and Morgan, Lincoln and Guba, etc.). Taken together, these represented the modern approach, following Francis Bacon's terminology.

Much progress certainly occurred in mathematics, and in the physical and social sciences (Augustin Cauchy, David Hilbert, Albert Einstein, Karl Popper, Imre Lakatos, Thomas Kuhn) but the means rapidly become more and more uncertain. As we have observed, Bacon's objectives were adopted, but his means were found to be unsatisfactory, and each successive writer on methodology (Francis Bacon, Mill, Whewell etc.) further complicated the proposed methodology in an effort to find a method that worked. Meantime, many scientific arguments have been shown to be flawed, many experiments have been faked, and it is hard to find any significant discovery that has genuinely followed from the careful use of any methodological precepts (Paul Feyerabend, Richard Rorty). Worse, we now have proofs that no universal method exists even for deciding if formal propositions are mutually consistent (Évariste Galois, Georg Cantor, Kurt Gödel, Alonso Church, Alan Turing), let alone accounting for observed reality even in the promising-looking physical sciences (Nils Bohr, Werner Heisenberg, Ilya Prigogine).

LIKELY STORIES AND THE POSTMODERN

An earlier section noted that in the late twentieth century there was a widespread acceptance of the methodological failure of Bacon's 'modern' approach. In our subsequent, 'postmodern' world, there is an inbuilt suspicion about universal truth, absolute reality, total objectivity etc. Nevertheless, those who nostalgically protest that 'without such certainties anything goes' certainly over-react.[3] The current practice, in almost all disciplines, is to continue with impersonal, quasi-objective writing wherever possible, and to invoke the soli-

---

[3] ' "Relativism" is the view that every belief on a certain topic, or perhaps about *any* topic, is as good as any other. No one holds this view. . . . The philosophers who get *called* "relativists" are those who say that the grounds for choosing such opinions are less algorithmic than had been thought.' (Rorty 1982b, p. 166).

darity of communities of like-minded researchers to select among competing stories. Since it has proved impossible to establish, by scientific means, *precisely* what people mean for even the simplest of utterances, methods that require absolute precision have fallen into disuse. Instead, in many disciplines people have rediscovered that their common language is that of natural speech. Information expressed in natural speech is as easy to exchange as natural speech, and no more difficult to understand.

The information technologist's tale is an example of one way of taking account of this postmodern context. The style of writing is impersonal, although there is an acceptance of diverse opinions in the area, even an unwillingness to define terms precisely. There appears to be a willingness to accept culture-based interpretations of some concepts at their face value, even where the cited quotations hint at disagreement under the surface. Although this tale contains something that looks suspiciously like a mathematical formula, it merely associates three postulated aspects to a desired outcome. Following some discussion as to what this might mean, the researchers construct a questionnaire to elicit 'importance measures', and the results are analysed to see if the answers agree with the expected model.

Although this methodology may seem rather loose, the findings are potentially useful for a number of purposes. The paper is likely to be read by IT professionals, who may be interested in knowing how other respondents rated the various factors in the model, in developing new products to help managers globalise their business, or in refining such models.

Moreover, for all of these purposes, the very imprecision of the approach is a positive advantage. In the 1970s it used to be thought that data, as processed by computers, was straightforward to deal with: it amounted to individual records of transactions, and was inherently value-free. Information, of the sort that managers wanted to deal with, was much more dependent on interpreta tion, on what went on inside managers' heads (Checkland 1981). Times have changed, and from today's perspectives on information systems, data has been found to be rather difficult to exchange: data aggregates are too dependent on categories and data models, whereas opinions and judgements of the sort found in the information technologist's tale are actually less problematic. There is a branch of media that caters for managers, and trends, dependencies, risks etc. are freely exchanged: this is evidence for a culture that values narratives of this general sort.

It seems therefore that, following the failure of the so-called 'modern' approach in the twentieth century, we stand at the beginning of the twenty-first with our fondness for the likely story intact, but with rather fewer of the pretensions of the scientific method. It is the modest purpose of this book to observe what some researchers do now, rather than attempt to prescribe what researchers should do.

Table 1.2 gives some pointers to the differing styles used in the stories in this collection. They share the academic narrative style described above.

Table 1.2. Some pointers to differing styles

Paper	The style of the story
Environmental geochemist (Chapter 3)	Identity of the writer: just the one reference: 'Over the past 5–6 years our studies . . .'. Contextual knowledge assumed: terminology, implicit methodology, statistical inference. Objectivity/truth claims: positivist standpoint adopted in quantitative conclusions about estuarine chemistry; no discussion of adequacy of sample or sample sites to support conclusions; otherwise generally avoids jumping to conclusions.
Mediarist (Chapter 8)	Identity of the writer: one full section devoted to an autobiographical report. Contextual knowledge assumed: that of a well-read consumer. Objectivity/truth claims: although apparently disavowed in the poems at the end, the conclusions are presented in ways the reader is invited to endorse.
Spiritual researcher (Chapter 11)	Identity of the writer: the writer hides behind the personification 'Spirited Scotland'. Contextual knowledge assumed: understanding of the social services in Scotland and devolved institutions. Objectivity/truth claims: realist standpoint adopted in talking about the requirements and intentions of these organisations; the conclusions merely that there is a need for these bodies to adopt the author's agenda.
Psychologist (Chapter 6)	Identity of the writer: very personal, giving an insight into the methods and excitement of research in this branch of cognitive psychology. Contextual knowledge assumed: intended for a popular audience, familiar with visual media and the difficulty of understanding unfamiliar speakers. Objectivity/truth claims: the experiments described are of the hypothetico-deductive kind, and numerous theories are outlined. None of these is claimed to be true. The conclusion is (modestly) that the research is of some value.
Anthropologist (Chapter 9)	Identity of the writer: considerable personal details, since the writer's values and culture are assumed to impact observation. Contextual knowledge assumed: general knowledge about hospitals and their procedures, familiarity with the species under observation. Objectivity/truth claims: data drawn from the personal stories of two interview subjects are used to corroborate theories in contemporary anthropological literature, and criticise directly and by implication the work of modernist anthropologists.
Marine biologist (Chapter 2)	Identity of the writer: appears only in the acknowledgement at the end. Contextual knowledge assumed: background on ecological issues, predator–prey cycles.

Table 1.2. *Continued*

Paper	The style of the story
	Objectivity/truth claims: hypothetico-deductive method. The paper puts forward a theory (parametric model) and its predictions are compared with data gathered by other researchers. However, no objectivity or truth claim is made beyond drawing attention to the goodness of fit.
Information technologist (Chapter 5)	Identity of the writer: the pronoun 'we' never refers to the author or the reader, but to various hypothetical groups of professionals. Contextual knowledge assumed: role of IT in business, business mix circa 2000. Objectivity/truth claims: hypothetico-deductive method applied to very qualitative survey-based research; conclusions asserted despite modest survey size.
Health policy researcher (Chapter 12)	Identity of the writer: considerable personal details, since the methodology involves the researcher's judgement and discrimination. Contextual knowledge assumed: the reader is expected to have a general understanding of the operation of the health service, and of cancer care. Objectivity/truth claims: similar to grounded theory, concerns are subjectively selected from edited transcripts of interviews with subjects; it is assumed the resulting summaries will prompt the consideration of policy changes.
Nurse philosopher (Chapter 10)	Identity of the writer: 'I suggest' repeatedly challenges evidence as objective. 'We' seems to refer to an imagined solidarity of health care professionals. Contextual knowledge assumed: assumes readership familiar with nursing practice. Objectivity/truth claims: a mechanistic nursing model is harmful.
Statistician (Chapter 4)	Identity of the writer: a (typical) practising consultant statistician. Contextual knowledge assumed: standard research methodology such as questionnaire construction. Objectivity/truth claims: data can be useless.
Political historian (Chapter 7)	Identity of the writer: a 1978 PhD in Czech political history. Contextual knowledge assumed: current affairs and the role of official media. Objectivity/truth claims: that historians inevitably impose their own views on intractable and complex events.
Chapter 1	Identity of the writer: the pronoun 'we' is used merely to include (co-opt) the reader. Contextual knowledge assumed: relationship of academics to academia. Objectivity/truth claims: hypothetico-deductive method; very small sample size leads to caution in statement of conclusions.

THE EVIDENCE OFFERED

The purpose of research remains to gather and analyse some evidence, in order to contribute towards a paradigm, or likely story, which might later be used to explain or predict something. A research paper presents the story of this gathering and analysis, seeking to persuade the reader that its conclusion can now be regarded as established; at least until it is refined by further research.

The reader is asked to consider the research objectives, the methods used in gathering evidence, the quality of the evidence itself, and the steps of the analysis and the force of the conclusions. Some fields of enquiry are more demanding than others, for example, forbidding publication until the end of the programme that has been outlined, or even until the findings have been accepted by a sufficient number of experts.

There are some fields of enquiry where certain kinds of evidence will simply not be accepted, no matter who the author is or how well the methodology is documented. For example, in setting their faces against explanations in terms of magic or paraphysics, the Royal Society also dismissed all similar-looking evidence, however well written, and this convention continues today. For example, the chemist William Crookes (1832–1919) became a president of the Royal Society, but nevertheless could present evidence of levitation in 1874:

> The most striking cases of levitation which I have witnessed have been with Mr Home. On three separate occasions have I seen him raised completely from the floor of the room. (Gjertsen 1989, p.196)

Crookes gives plenty of detailed scientifically recorded evidence, and is an eminent witness. But we cannot accept the evidence. Even the words Crookes uses seem to imply that there may be something special about the circumstances (Mr Home, his room), or the observer, and we suspect an illusion or fabrication.

On the other hand, for example, sailors' tales of gigantic waves, previously dismissed by the scientific community, have suddenly received backing from direct satellite observation (Maxwave 2002). Naturally, there are mathematical theories at hand to make such tales, derided for centuries, suddenly acceptable. Marine insurers now have to take into account 30-metre waves as a common occurrence in calm seas, even in the absence of adverse currents.

If the research communities have declined to perform an analysis of their own methodology in rejecting or accepting contributions, their critics have not been slow to do so. Feyerabend, Kuhn and Polanyi all find it hard to see much rigour or system in such differing treatment of what looks on the face of it to be similar evidence, and conclude that it is ultimately the belief system of the researcher (or the critical reader) that is at issue.

LIKELY STORIES AS NARRATIVE

Rorty (1982a, p. 202), having argued that objectivity and scientific method in quantitative subjects are illusory, turns to social science:

If we get rid of traditional notions of 'objectivity' and 'scientific method' we shall be able to see the social sciences as continuous with literature – as interpreting other people to us, and thus enlarging and deepening our sense of community. . . . If we emphasise this side of their achievement, . . . we shall not worry about how this style is related to the 'galilean' style which 'quantified behavioural science' has tried to emulate.

What happens when we view the research paper as literature? The opening sentence of a narrative normally takes pains to introduce the central character immediately, if occasionally indirectly, as with:

Hale knew, before he had been in Brighton three hours, that they meant to murder him.

Here, the central characters are contained in the 'they', but the context (in Graham Greene's *Brighton Rock*) is already clear: a criminal gang in Brighton.

The central character in fiction is not always a human being: it may for example be a place or an event. In research writing, the opening sentence of the narrative generally places the research topic centre stage. In the health policy researcher's tale, the opening sentence is:

This chapter will describe and reflect on the development of recording individuals' experience, in a research context, as a method of improving health and social care.

Although people and their experiences (evidently to be viewed from their angle) are placed centre stage, they are not the main characters in this narrative: they are mere stereotypes, much as in other forms of narrative, where many of the characters are also stock fictions, such as the *fall guy*, the *constant wife* etc.: here we have the *patient*, the *health care provider*. It is relatively rare for the actual people or the researchers who provide the detail for these stereotypes to be introduced at all. Also, we are left at this stage to form our own hypotheses about the nature of the difference in experience, guided by the sentences which immediately follow. In Atkinson's paper these encourage us to focus on the effect of remote treatment on the lives of people being treated for life-threatening disease: a category of patient, a category of treatment, and a category of experience, to be viewed from the two sides, patient and health care provider. However, in this case the reader is assumed to be already familiar with the health care provider's viewpoint and so the experiences related are all of patients.

Atkinson's paper consists of several threads of narrative. First, there is the impersonal narrative of the research task itself, how it builds on past stereotypes from previous research, and collects stories from patients and tentatively draws up conclusions and stereotypes to influence policy. Second, there are the personal stories of each of the subjects that are depicted separately in a narrative form, once a shared set of circumstances (the hospital, geography, illness, and policies concerning treatment) has been outlined. The hope in presenting these stories is that the researchers will be able to communicate the 'understanding and perceptions people have of their own world', and so the researchers consciously sought common themes from sentences they recorded in interview diaries. The researchers hope these notes and themes are not distorted by the lens of an external theory. On the other hand, they decide in advance that many aspects of the patient's story such as social background and circumstances are irrelevant, and deliberately ignore them in both note-taking and thematic analysis, beyond a pre-screening of the sample for age, gender or illness bias.

The aim of the researchers is to develop paradigmatic conflations of some aspects of these stories: 'to present a story that has created a change of the researcher's perception (a paradigm shift) or knowledge'. Such paradigms, like the effect of superposed facial images, are in literal terms myths or fictions, but may offer tentative generalisations just as the superposed images may result in some observations on average characteristics. The significance of any piece of evidence in this study, however, was weighted not by frequency of occurrence but by the 'importance assigned by the individuals'.

Critics of such methods can justifiably object that while the researchers may aim to avoid the lens of an external theory, cultural distortions are inevitable. For example, patients readily absorb the descriptive categories of their doctors etc., which might create themes that would otherwise not have emerged. Also, the choice of categories to ignore already implies certain theoretical predispositions.

Atkinson's paper outlines the method and then gives us an account of the themes distilled from the interviews, which, as promised, strip away all circumstantial detail, no doubt partly in the interests of patient anonymity. In the anthropologist's tale, by contrast, the interview subject's hobby and its associated value system are carefully analysed: they would probably have been rejected in Atkinson's study as irrelevant and not recorded. However, the anthropologist's tale may correspond better to the interview notes for just one of Atkinson's subjects; Rapport merely hazards some notes that might represent common themes were they to surface in other interviews.

In the end, we are back with *Timaeus*, thinking about what we would accept as a likely story. In any community, we are more likely to accept an account that seems consistent with conventional wisdom (possibly enhancing, extending, or partly explaining it). When some evidence appears to challenge the conventional wisdom, it may take some time for the Kuhnian 'scientific revolution' of discovery to take place. In some cases such a difficult discovery may illuminate some other problem. For example, if everyday cooking processes with temperatures higher than 125°C produce industrially significant levels of the carcinogen acrylamide, might it help to explain the increasing incidence of cancer during the twentieth century as these cooking processes became more widely used?

Table 1.3 indicates aspects of the sort of evidence offered in each of our research papers.

Table 1.3. Types of evidence

Paper	Evidence offered
Environmental geochemist (Chapter 3)	Choice of sample: mud samples taken at particular places in the Clyde estuary. Choice of observations: chemical analyses following treatment of mud. Paradigms offered: observations on this estuary at this time may correlate with other estuaries or times, depending on such matters as industrial history: the mythical estuary and the mythical pollution scenario.
Mediarist (Chapter 8)	Choice of sample: BBC as offering a conservative ideological stance, other media chosen for typifying attitudes to the monarchy. Choice of observations: comments on the message conveyed. Paradigms offered: perceptions of distinctive role of monarchy in the UK: the mythical monarch and the mythical commoner.
Spiritual researcher (Chapter 11)	Choice of sample: samples of writings on policy. Choice of observations: spiritual aspects of health care. Paradigms offered: proposals for directions of social policy that might be adopted elsewhere: the mythical policy-maker.
Psychologist (Chapter 6)	Choice of sample: samples of psychological research. Choice of observations: evolution of theories and hypotheses. Paradigms offered: the McGurk effect presented as a well-known phenomenon.
Anthropologist (Chapter 9)	Choice of sample: extended interviews with two hospital porters. Choice of observations: what they say about their job and their colleagues. Paradigms offered: some support given to existing paradigms of a mythical work culture.
Marine biologist (Chapter 2)	Choice of sample: data taken from research papers, selected by subject matter. Choice of observations: how well they fit with a suitably parameterised model. Paradigms offered: explicit quantitative predictive model tentatively offered for test: a new myth.
Information technologist (Chapter 5)	Choice of sample: some respondents to a survey, selected by convenience. Choice of observations: their attitudes to IT as enabling technology. Paradigms offered: explicit hypotheses predicting relative success of enterprises: a new myth of enterprise.
Health policy researcher (Chapter 12)	Choice of sample: some cancer patients from rural communities, selected by availability. Choice of observations: their views on their treatment. Paradigms offered: we are left with the feeling that many patients would respond similarly to the sample: a new mythical patient.

Table 1.3. *Continued*

Paper	Evidence offered
Nurse philosopher (Chapter 10)	Choice of sample: none. Some anecdotes from referenced material. Choice of observations: none. Paradigms offered: two myths: repeatable controlled trials versus the nurse experience.
Statistician (Chapter 4)	Choice of sample: a specific survey on leisure activities in Kilbarchan. Choice of observations: discussions that influenced the sources of data. Paradigms offered: two myths: statisticians that can help researchers.
Political historian (Chapter 7)	Choice of sample: revisit the sources of the PhD thesis with additional hindsight. Choice of observations: naturally focuses on sources of historical error. Paradigms offered: the myth of the historian's struggle towards objectivity and truth.
Chapter 1	Choice of sample: some research papers. Probably haphazard or accidental grouping. Choice of observations: allegedly based on historical concerns of researchers. Paradigms offered: explicit hypotheses on how to write (or read) research papers (the mythical reader and the mythical researcher).

THE ACADEMIC COMMUNITY

For Francis Bacon and his circle the creation of a suitable academic community was indispensable. It was realised well after Bacon's death with the foundation of the Royal Society and similar bodies in other countries. Fortunately for the project, universities quickly (re)established themselves as principal suppliers and hosts of academic communities, and this situation has continued to the present day.

The academic community provides the cultural continuity that is a prerequisite of Bacon's programme. It provides a forum for debate and the exposition of knowledge, as today at research conferences, for training of research students, and for examination and review.

THE RESEARCH CYCLE

It is natural that some participants in the community have identified cyclical processes of discovery and analysis. We have already reviewed the hermeneu-

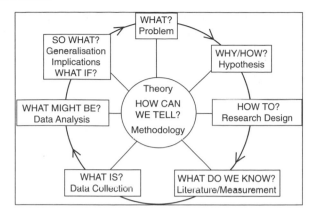

Figure 1.2. The Research Cycle. (Adapted from Frankfort-Nachmias and Nachmias, 1992).

tic circle and hints at Kuhn's scientific revolutions. Let us now consider the intermediate size of cycle where a particular research idea is taken up, developed, and the findings analysed: this is yet another cycle of evolution (Figure 1.2).

> In short, the process of research consists of deciding **why** we want to research **what** we want to research, and **how** we think we are going to do it (the planning phase). Subsequently, we decide **how to** actually do the research and then **do** it (what data we will collect and how, and then what we will do with these data when we have got them). Finally, we present the results of our efforts. Now, as a result of our research, we think we know something which was not known before, and so are in a position to ask and answer the question: **so what?** (Harvey, n.d.)

The cycle identified by Harvey is very similar to that of Francis Bacon, and corresponds to an evolutionary cycle of the likely story. The approach of Frankfort-Nachmias and Nachmias referred to in Figure 1.2 has been viewed as old-fashioned and overly empiricist in using the words 'Data Collection' and 'Data Analysis' but data does not have to be positivist or quantitative to be analysed: our sample papers are full of evidence and analysis, and not all are from the positivist tradition.

LIKELY STORIES AND THE ACADEMIC COMMUNITY

In the above quotations it would seem that the word 'we' refers to an academic community, in historical descent from Plato's school of Athens: a group of thinkers discussing research problems of common interest. With the fragmentation of knowledge into different disciplines, portions of any such academic community meet at focused conferences at which knowledge in a particular discipline will be presented and discussed.

As we have seen, what stories are regarded as likely is partly a question of prevailing custom (or culture). The evolution of likely stories seems to be as a result of addressing new aspects of a problem, gathering further results, performing further analysis, drawing further conclusions, or applying new critical methods. From today's standpoint such evolution always seems to be an improvement: from mythology to science, from ignorance to knowledge, from mistaken notions to better ones etc. But we know that evolution will mean today's standpoint will probably seem ignorant and mistaken when viewed from tomorrow.

It is not hard to find other writers taking this view of likely stories. A simple web search (in 2002) turned up the following:

(a) Ross Lee Graham: 'Status of Logic in Science-Systems' (Graham 1994)

LIKELY STORIES. The impetus to create likely stories has never been adequately explained. Ingenious minds early set themselves to inquire how experience is to be accounted for. Intellectual history is regarded by some scholars as a history of development from mythology to science.

Some ground of justification or explanation is thought of, i.e., a likely story that seems to account for an experience and seems to reconcile it with the current state of beliefs. Sometimes a description is given of an occurrence but its likely story, the story that accounts for it, changes. With time, different stories evolve that become more effective in their applications, displacing those with less power. A kind of 'natural' selection occurs here. Then the understanding adapts itself to the new story that has been found for explanation, and the description receives a new life and in time the description gets modified to fit the new story better. This series of events is exemplified in the genesis of celestial mechanics. For example, this kind of change in explanation is shown in part by Kepler's kinematics laws of planetary motion. Kepler's explanation was displaced by Newton's explanation. Another example, the Lorentz transformation, a description (empirical); Lorentz's explanation was displaced by Einstein's, etc.

(b) David M. Mills: 'Dimensions of Embodiment' (Mills 1996)

Observation – we observe some phenomena of interest, gather and attempt to interpret our observations. (Note that even our most basic observations are conditioned by our prior habits of perception and our earlier theories.)

. . .

Since observation is both the first and last step in the procedure, the scientific method is an endless cycle of exploration rather than any kind of completed package, and the process results not in an ever-rising pile of fragments of 'truth,' but rather in a series of constructed theories that are ever more effective approximations to truth, what Plato called 'likely stories.' This situation is what Kelly calls 'constructive alternativism' as he characterizes it in 'The Psychology of the Unknown.'

Our venture as scientists, then is not to press with one hand on what is presumed to be known for sure and reach out with the other into the unknown for more bits of the puzzle, but rather to proceed from propositions which are admittedly faulty, in the hope that we can complete fully the experiential cycles which will enable us to formulate new propositions that are perhaps less faulty.

THE PERSISTENCE OF THE ACADEMIC COMMUNITY

As with Socrates, members of such a community frequently place a value on such academic discussion well above their own, and try to preserve an intellectual honesty despite pressures from national or vested interests. Over the centuries, governments and religious authorities have tried to censor such inquiring movements; but the tradition has continued down the centuries. Perpetuating the academe is our duty as academics: our reward is the enjoyment of intellectual debate and discovery.

Table 1.4 indicates the role of the research question and contribution to knowledge in each of the papers considered.

Table 1.4. The role of the research question

Paper	Academic community matters
Environmental geochemist (Chapter 3)	Nature of the research community: researchers into environmental chemistry and ecology. Research question: recovery of estuaries from industrial pollution. New knowledge: new data of interest to other researchers in predicting ecological behaviour.
Mediarist (Chapter 8)	Nature of the research community: media studies researchers and their students. Research question: whether relationship between cultural history and media content is just a figment of academic discourse. New knowledge: conclusions from media studies were not challenged on methodological grounds despite debate beyond academic communities.
Spiritual researcher (Chapter 11)	Nature of the research community: (spiritual pressure groups?) Research question: how to promote a spiritual focus in health policy. New knowledge: some suggested conceptual analogies to help get the message across.
Psychologist (Chapter 6)	Nature of the research community: cognitive psychologists. Research question: explanation of McGurk effect. New knowledge: impact on theories of perception.
Anthropologist (Chapter 9)	Nature of the research community: anthropologists. Research question: exploring how other people live. New knowledge: insights into roles, employee cultures.

Table 1.4. *Continued*

Paper	Academic community matters
Marine biologist (Chapter 2)	Nature of the research community: zoologists. Research question: what mathematical models can be used as predictors? New knowledge: some suggested models which fit with some past data.
Information technologist (Chapter 5)	Nature of the research community: management and IT researchers. Research question: how can the IT infrastructures to support strategic management be improved? New knowledge: some suggestions for how improvements in awareness etc. can be achieved.
Health policy researcher (Chapter 12)	Nature of the research community: health studies. Research question: improving health service procedures in dealing with seriously ill rural patients. New knowledge: may encourage health professionals to take patients' needs more into account.
Nurse philosopher (Chapter 10)	Nature of the research community: nursing practitioners as distinct from pharmaceutical researchers. Research question: the value and meaning of 'evidence-based medicine'. New knowledge: nursing care is more important.
Statistician (Chapter 4)	Nature of the research community: all quantitative researchers. Research question: the value of statistical analysis before data collection. New knowledge: new for non-statisticians perhaps.
Political historian (Chapter 7)	Nature of the research community: fellow historians. Research question: the nature of historical dispassion. New knowledge: some new factual detail, and further examples of how even serious historians can be misled by what they want to believe.
Chapter 1	Nature of the research community: academic staff in universities. Research question: what is characteristic of research? New knowledge: a possible set of criteria, expressed in somewhat loose terms.

CONCLUSIONS

A tentative conclusion from the above is that much if not all academic research follows in spirit and even in general form the research programme (re)inaugurated by Francis Bacon, characterised by the journey of discovery, the offering of evidence, the scholarly style and the academic community. We offer this overview and the associated research papers as a celebration of the unity of the academic tradition, while recognising that many conflicting methodologies, epistemologies and ontologies, and not a few controversies, lurk within.

REFERENCES

Bacon, F. (2000) *The Instauratio Magna: Last Writings*, ed. trans G. Rees. Oxford University Press, Oxford (first published 1620).

Checkland, P. B. (1981) *Systems Theory, Systems Practice.* John Wiley & Sons, Chichester.

Chladenius, J. M. (1988) *Einleitung zur richtigen Auslegung vernünftiger Reden und Schriften*, trans. D. Mueller-Vollmer. In K. Mueller-Vollmer (ed.) *The Hermeneutics Reader* (pp. 54–71). Continuum, New York (first published 1742).

Crowe, M. K. (1996) Heraclitus and information systems. *Computing and Information Systems* **3**, 95–106.

Frankfort-Nachmias, C., Nachmias, D. (1992) *Research Methods in the Social Sciences.* Edward Arnold, London.

Gjertsen, D. (1989) *Science and Philosophy: Past and Present.* Penguin, Harmondsworth.

Glaser, B., Strauss, A. L. (1967) *The Discovery of Grounded Theory: Strategies for Qualititative Research.* Aldine de Gruyter, New York.

Graham, R. L. (1994) Status of logic in science-systems. Available at: www.rosslg.com/works/WebNotes/Systems/sciencesystems.html. Accessed January 2006.

Harvey, D. (n.d.) AEF801: What do we mean by research? Available at: www.staff.ncl.ac.uk/david.harvey/AEF801/What.html. Accessed January 2006.

Kuhn, T. (1962) *The Structure of Scientific Revolutions.* University of Chicago Press, Chicago, IL.

Kuhn, T. S. (1992) *The Copernican Revolution: Planetary Astronomy in the Development of Western Thought.* MUF Books.

Maxwave (2002) EU project EVK:3-2000-00544. Available at: w3g.gkss.de/projects/maxwave. Accessed January 2006.

Mead, M. (1928) *Coming of Age in Samoa: A Psychological Study of Primitive Youth for Western Civilization.* William Morrow, New York.

Mills, D. M. (1996) Dimensions of embodiment: towards a conversational science of human action, part 2. Available at: www.ati-net.com/articles/mills2.php. Accessed January 2006.

Plato (1965) *Timaeus and Critias*, trans Desmond Lee. Penguin Books.

Rorty, R. (1982a) Method, social science, and social hope. In *Consequences of Pragmatism: Essays 1972–1980* (pp. 191–210). Harvester Wheatsheaf, Hemel Hempstead.

Rorty, R. (1982b) Pragmatism, relativism, and irrationalism. In *Consequences of Pragmatism: Essays 1972–1980* (pp. 160–175). Harvester Wheatsheaf, Hemel Hempstead.

Rorty, R. (1982c) The world well lost. In *Consequences of Pragmatism: Essays 1972–1980* (pp. 3–18). Harvester Wheatsheaf, Hemel Hempstead.

Whewell, W. (1837) *History of the Inductive Sciences.* Republished in Butts, R. E. (ed.) (1989) *William Whewell: Theory of Scientific Method.* Hackett, Indianapolis, IN.

2 Studying Complexity: Are We Approaching the Limits of Science?

IAN BOYD

Sea Mammal Research Unit, University of St Andrews, UK

INTRODUCTION

This contribution to a book about approaches to research is directed less towards the science I am undertaking and more towards the challenges that exist to commonly held notions in science. During my career I have had the pleasure of studying several specialisations in biology, including endocrinology, animal energetics, behavioural ecology and ecosystem science. This is a very wide range but all of these fields have a strong underlying common theme: they are all different ways of approaching the problem of complexity. Like many scientists, I have spent my time taking a very small part of a big problem and understanding that thoroughly in the hope that, some day, we will use that to build a better understanding of the greater whole. However, with the benefit of hindsight, perhaps I have done too little to connect the various fields of study, and this chapter is a way of beginning that process.

One of the criticisms I have heard of science is that too much of it is geared to understanding more and more about less and less. My standard riposte is that, so long as the details illustrate general underlying principles, this is a desirable route to follow. But I have to confess that my riposte is sometimes less than full-blooded because I am aware that there is more than a grain of truth in the criticism. I then comfort myself further by suggesting that a great deal of science is actually a part of the process of training both the individual and the community. Training the community comes in the form of adding to the body of documented knowledge, however trivial that contribution may at first appear (although much of this knowledge might not emerge well from a narrowly-based cost–benefit analysis). The training of individuals is a process that continues throughout scientific careers and, as science becomes increasingly technically demanding, a greater proportion of a scientist's time could be put down to training. The issue is that it is not recognised as such.

Interdisciplinary Research: Diverse Approaches in Science, Technology, Health and Society.
Edited by J. Atkinson and M. Crowe.

My own desire has always been to attempt to synthesise general principles from narrowly founded information. But I have found that this requires more than the talents contained within a single individual. For this to occur effectively science must become teamwork and, consequently, the rate of scientific progress is governed to an extent by the sociology of teams and the efficiency with which intellectual understanding is exchanged. Forming effective teams is not something scientists are trained to do and it is not something they generally understand. A problem that many scientists face is that they are studying processes that have complex behaviour while they are themselves set within a complex environment. Unless we solve for both simultaneously, we will not solve some of the biggest problems facing humanity.

In this chapter I will explore what I believe is one of the biggest problems facing biology. This problem is *complexity*. A fledgling field known as *complexity science* is beginning to emerge. *Complexity* is a feature that is common to issues beyond biology. I have already mentioned its connection with sociology but it is important in understanding issues from business operations to financial markets and weather forecasting. Physicists are also grappling with the problem of complexity. However, I believe it is within biology that the greatest challenges may lie. Complexity has application right across the field from genomics to ecosystem science, and I believe that biologists in general are poorly equipped to deal with its consequences. In fact, some may even deny its existence.

Complexity occurs where the behaviour of a system cannot be predicted from the sum of its parts. Increasingly we see systems, such as ecosystems or a large-scale business operation, as having emergent properties that could not be predicted from detailed knowledge of their components. This is also sometimes known as *self-organised criticality*, which is a term familiar in chaos theory. Nevertheless, we know that complex systems are not chaotic but they may be on the verge of chaos. In nature, as well as in the business world, systems that are chaotic will not survive long but it is possible that the systems that survive best are those that are complex and are on the edge of chaos. This is because these are the systems that respond most flexibly to external challenges.

In physics, *complexity* can be expressed as the disconnection between the known world of particles and their interactions between one another, and the world that these particles are built into. No physical theory predicts the existence of teapots or other esoteric objects and yet they are a part of the way in which the physical world is organised and they are bound by the same physical laws as the fundamental components that form physical matter (Ellis 2005). Similarly, organisms are physically based but there is little hope of predicting all aspects of an organism's biology from first principles.

I suspect that, when faced with a complex problem, most biologists would respond by suggesting that more research is required. As an editor of a science journal and as a member of international science committees, whose roles are mainly to provide advice based on a synthesis of relevant science, I have always been uncomfortable with this type of conclusion to a study. In some cases this conclusion may well be valid but more often the problem being investigated cannot be solved by investigating more and more detail.

THE NATURE OF COMPLEXITY

By the definition given above, complexity is the study of the behaviour of systems. In this case, a system is any group of interacting components (sometimes also known as agents) around which there is a clearly defined boundary between it and the rest of the world. There are also clearly definable inputs from the world to the system that cross the boundary and, similarly, there are outputs. The best way to visualise this is to view an individual organism as a system.

Although complexity could be seen as a field in its own right, it emerges out of the need to reconcile two opposing processes in science. One involves the drive for reductionism, where the view is that big problems, like how the universe works, are simply the sum of its parts and, if one can understand the fundamental parts, one can then understand the operation of the whole system of interest. Conversely, there is the effort to reconstruct systems from their component parts, which could be described as post-reductionism (*sensu* post-genomics).

Flaws in this process of system engineering begin to appear pretty quickly with the increasing complexity of the system one is studying. If one has a system composed of just two simple components there is clearly the possibility for each of the components only to have a relationship with one other component. But as the number of components increases, the number of interactions each individual can have will increase as a geometric series described by $(n^2 - n)/2$. This means that by the time there are 5 components in the system, the number of interactions has grown to 10, and for a system containing 10 components the number will be 45. Moreover, if the components are not simple and have the capability of modifying the strength or quality of their interactions as a result of their state then the total number of possible interactions increases in proportion to the number of states. Added to this, one also has to take into account the state of the observer, in this case the scientist himself, who will have a specific interaction with the different components and may not be able to observe some components or even be aware of their existence.

This may all seem a little detached and esoteric, but it is the essence of complexity. Small, seemingly understandable two-way interactions between two components of a system, which can often be studied and thoroughly understood in isolation, cannot be easily summed to predict the behaviour of whole systems. This is not just because it is sometimes impossible completely to characterise the interactions between all the components, but also because the state of an interaction between two components depends on the presence of other components of the system, even though they may not have anything directly to do with the interaction concerned.

Part of my science career was spent studying the endocrinology of seasonal reproduction in mammals. The interactions between hormones in the body are a good illustration of a complex system and also of the inadequacy of the techniques that I, and others at that time, were applying to the understanding of reproductive endocrinology in animals, including humans. The standard methods used controlled experiments in which one factor was varied while keeping others constant. Observations were made of the effects of this treatment upon levels of circulating hormones. In their most complex forms, one might have varied two or three factors (such as light, temperature and the level of a particular hormone) simultaneously but these multifactorial experiments very quickly begin to become too large to handle because of all the control groups that are required. These experiments produced an understanding of the covariance of particular hormones under specific sets of circumstances but it proved to be impossible to understand from these experiments how the whole system operated. There was too much uncertainty in the results and there was no way of connecting the response observed under one set of circumstances with the response under another set. Moreover, we knew that there were other hormones involved in determining responses that we could not measure so we were blind to part of the system being studied. I recall the long discussions with colleagues, often in the local pub, about the next experiment to do. One colleague even named his experiments after the pub in which they were invented. There was an incremental progression of understanding but I was usually left feeling that the key to success was a long way off and perhaps unachievable.

Part of the problem of complexity is the mindset of the observer. I am sure that I and my colleagues studying seasonal reproduction thought there would turn out to be one important key interaction or hormone that tended to exercise overall control of the process we were studying. I see this repeated in the field of community ecology, where the concept of 'keystone species' in ecosystems has been invented. In this case, community ecologists are searching for key species within ecosystems, the dynamics of which are largely driven by these key species. Although there may be some ecosystems in which certain species tend to dominate (and some physiological processes which are dominated by particular hormones), I believe the concept of the *key* to the dynamics of a system is largely an attempt by the observer to rationalise a complex problem in a way that makes it tractable within the norms of scientific procedure. However, this does not mean the process of investigation that follows brings us any nearer to a solution. Complex systems simply cannot be rationalised in this way.

An easy way to visualise a complex system is using social groups as an example. I experienced this when arriving to spend the summer on an isolated Antarctic station that had been occupied by only three people for the previous six months. Being the first injection of a new face for such a long time always resulted in social readjustments. Two individuals can build a particular relationship that may be stable but adding a third into the relationship can change the stable state of the original two-way interaction. Adding further individuals can lead to even more changes and may cause instability between some individuals. This is described more formally in Box 2.1.

Box 2.1. Illustration from a model complex system of how small changes in the system can have effects that range well beyond those involving the individual components directly affected by the change

The results of the interactions between the components of a system can be expressed as the sum of two matrices, the matrix of interaction **M** and the matrix of association **A**, with the vector of individual states **s**. In **M**, the value of an interaction i that is neutral is unity but $0 < i < 2$. In **A**, the sum of all associations between any component and all other components is unity, which assumes that each component has a finite capacity to form associations and that it divides its total capacity between the components of the system. For individuals in a social structure, this level of association could be dictated by the spatial spread of individuals. Therefore, applying the matrices **M** and **A** to **s** through time produces an evolution of states through time for each component of the system. This is illustrated in Figure 2.1.

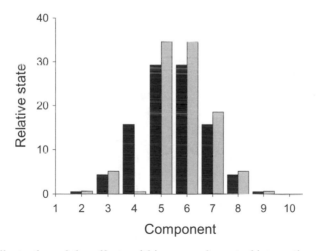

Figure 2.1. Illustration of the effects within a complex set of interactions of changing the strength of just one of the interactions in a matrix involving 10 components when all other interactions are neutral. This shows the consequences that changing the strength of ~1% of interactions can have for the state of all the components in the system. The black bars are the states before the change when all interactions are neutral and the grey bars are the states of components after the change in one interaction involving components 4 and 3.

The illustration in Figure 2.1 is built upon a simple simulation of a system of interacting components. It is possible to derive very complex behaviours for the components in a system from a simple set of rules. Chaotic behaviour is the most extreme of these. The problem being faced by scientists working on complex systems is that the only observations available are often the behaviour of some selected components of the system (as in the example from endocrinology given above). Given this information, is it possible to derive the rules being followed by the interacting components and, from this knowledge, is it then possible to predict the future behaviour of the system by knowing the starting conditions?

Unfortunately, in most natural cases it is not currently possible to predict behaviour of most normal systems, even if the rules are known. In Figure 2.1 for example, it would be very difficult to understand that the change observed in the state of component 7 was caused by a non-neutral interaction between components 4 and 5 if only component 7 was being observed. Thus, predictions of the stock market are not feasible and predictions of weather patterns are only feasible over the short term. Predictions about how ecosystems are likely to function in future are similarly infected by uncertainty.

Mathematicians and physicists are trained to describe systems using differential equations. These can be powerful tools for describing the dynamics of systems and the way in which components interact, but, while they can simulate complex behaviour, they are limited in their scope to solve the behaviour for its component parts. In my experience, mathematics is quite limited in its capacity to unravel complexity where it exists. The systems of equations required to achieve this quickly become too difficult to solve. Consequently, understanding the complex behaviour of systems is perhaps the greatest intellectual challenge faced by mankind. We can probably survive without being able to predict the weather or the stock market but I am less certain if mankind can survive without being able to manage the life support systems of the planet or the way in which genes interact to produce functioning organisms.

Since the discovery of DNA we have seen inexorable progress toward the understanding of how genetics works, and this has culminated in the documentation of whole genomes, including the human genome. However, the post-genomics era involves the reversal of the arrow of progress from reductionism to reconstruction. Bioinformatics has grown as an important tool for achieving the reconstruction as a result of the sum of the parts. As we set out on this quest, there are grand claims made about finding drugs to switch genes on and off to treat diseases based upon the assumption that there is a simple cause–effect relationship between gene activity and the function of their products. Unfortunately, I suspect it may turn out to be a lot more complex in many critical cases. Like the example given in Figure 2.1, switching on and off genes is likely to affect the activity of other components of the system in such a way as to produce some alarming side effects. Some early gene therapy is already beginning to show these types of unpredictable effects, and, when applying genetic engineering to the food we eat, it is wise to be cautious about the consequences for the environment. Complexity has a habit of coming back to hit us in ways that we could never predict.

In the case of ecosystems, we already know about the consequences of management. It is a popular belief that when there is some form of negative consequence of management in an ecosystem, such as harvesting natural populations, growing or felling forests or draining marshlands, these consequences are avoidable. In some cases, the consequences are indeed avoidable. Clearly, if one drains the water out of a marsh it will dry up, causing the components within the marshland ecosystem to decline, but the effects of fishing for one species compared to another are not so clear. We have a tendency to attempt to manage only small parts of whole ecosystems, such as a specific fish population, and then to ignore the effects that fish harvests may have in apparently remote parts of the ecosystem. As in the illustration in Figure 2.1, changing one component of the ecosystem can result in changes to all other components. Moreover, it is almost impossible to predict changes that are removed from the immediate interactions involving the exploited species, and even in the case of the exploited species themselves, much of the evidence suggests that we are not very good at predicting their populations.

The problems of studying complexity are magnified further when they are scaled up from ecosystems to the *Earth system*. In this case, the Earth system is the biosphere in which we and all other life exist. It is a system with potentially highly complex behaviour. If the Earth system is like the simpler systems already described, and there is no reason to believe that it is not, then we can expect to have very low power to predict what will happen as a result of changes to different components. Thus, our predictions of the effects of global warming are a best guess but how many people would be willing to bet their livelihoods on the predictions being correct? In reality, the complexity of the Earth system is such that we cannot predict what global warming will do to our world. If we cannot predict the dynamics of fish populations under reasonably controlled levels of exploitation, we certainly will never be able to predict the dynamics of the Earth system.

STUDYING COMPLEXITY: FROM THE REAL WORLD TO DAISIES AND BACK AGAIN

At the beginning of their book *The Ecological Detective*, Ray Hilborn and Marc Mangel (1997) quote from a friend faced with explaining to a complete stranger what it is that he does. Their friend is an ecologist of sorts. He attempts to draw a parallel between what he does and the more familiar activity of a detective trying to solve a crime. Little pieces of information are tested against an idea that explains how they might all fit together in a consistent way. A judgement, usually using some form of statistics, is made about the degree to which the idea (the hypothesis) is explained by the information (the data). This is a familiar process to many scientists.

However, the *idea* can be expressed in many different ways. Traditionally, hypothesis generation and testing has been the engine house of science, but where complex systems are concerned, a different approach may be necessary. As I have said, it is not possible, by definition, to understand a complex system by building up one's understanding by looking at small parts.

Nevertheless, modelling could provide us with a clue to the nature of complexity, even if it is quite a long way from allowing us to understand and predict the behaviour of complex systems. In this context, a model is a hypothesis that is a best-guess but highly simplified approximation of the real world. The example given in Box 2.1 was a model of an imaginary complex system.

Daisyworld is a model of the world constructed by James Lovelock (1992), the inventor of the *Gaia hypothesis*, as a response to claims of teleology levelled at the hypothesis. It is highly simplified, involving only two types of daisy, a black type and a white type. It attempts to demonstrate how life could modify the physical nature of an imaginary and simplified planet through the interaction of its biotic and physical features. The model shows a considerable degree of planetary temperature regulation is possible because of the presence of daisies with extremely simple biology.

This initial result has been expanded greatly by adding small but measured amounts of complexity that includes the capacity of the daisies to mutate into different colours. It also includes a degree of heterogeneity of heat transport to the surface of the planet brought on by planetary curvature (Ackland et al. 2003). These simple but realistic changes led to two important insights that were counter-intuitive and could not have been predicted except by simulation. The first of these is that whereas intuition might have suggested that daisies of specific colours would have been selected as the optimum for different environments, it was found that clumps of different coloured plants combined to regulate the temperature. Contrary to the reductionist, it is the system as a whole that is subject to natural selection and not the individual organisms as predicted by Darwinian theory.

The second insight is that, when exposed to radiation levels above a critical value, a desert was formed across a large area of the planet. The change in the daisies happened over a very small change in the level of radiation and suggested that there were critical features of this simple system that could result in catastrophic changes in its response. This has interesting parallels in what happens in the real world. We see these apparent non-linearities in responses of one component of a system to changes in another component, and this type of change could have been responsible for the last Ice Age and will almost certainly lead to the next one.

NON-LINEARITIES

Although the results of the very simple simulation presented in Figure 2.1 can suggest complex behaviour, that is far from the end of the story of complexity. The simulation contained no explicit non-linearities in the relationships between its components. In the Daisyworld model, the non-linearities emerged as natural features of the simple interaction between the daisies and their physical environment. The concept of non-linearity is illustrated further in Figure 2.2, which shows how an animal population might respond to changes in its food supply.

In this case, as food supply declines the population of animals shows little response, but once the food supply declines below a specific level, the population responds in an increasingly severe way. This type of non-linear response occurs because individual animals can pursue different strategies to maintain themselves under different levels of food supply. These strategies involve different forms of food storage, metabolic responses to starvation and changes in behaviour such as migration, cessation of reproduction or employing different hunting tactics. All these strategies can be applied to human and non-human animals. In general, the more advanced the animal, the greater will be the buffering capacity. Therefore, for man, we have systems of food delivery to areas of the world where there is food shortage and this increases the buffering capacity of the population to local declines in the food supply. However, we also know that the cusp of the non-linearity will become sharper the more buffering there is in the population, so that, should food delivery systems fail, the effects will be catastrophic.

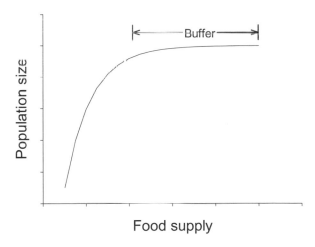

Figure 2.2. Schematic representation of the response of an animal population to changes in its food supply.

The consequence of this type of response of populations to changes in food supply for the management of ecosystems is that it is very easy to become lulled into a false sense of security by the buffering capacity of animal populations. This is the type of process that leads to the collapse of fisheries and that also leads to sudden flips in the structure of ecosystems, where, in as little as a few years in the case of dynamic marine ecosystems, the ecosystem can shift from being dominated by one group of species to dominance by another.

Adding non-linearities to the simple model illustrated in Figure 2.1 would probably take the model closer to the behaviour of the components within a real system but the results would be even more dynamic and unpredictable than before.

DIFFERENT TYPES OF COMPLEX MODELS

The Daisyworld model began as an exploration of the mechanisms that might lead to biological regulation of the temperature of a planet. It was both mechanistic and deterministic. This means that it attempted to include realistic values for physical and biological variables and realistic reaction norms[1] for the relationships between them. It also means that the result of the model will be the same however often the model is run. Unfortunately, this is not in itself a realistic situation. The world is not a deterministic system. Instead, many processes are seen to be stochastic, meaning that their outcomes are uncertain within specified boundaries and according to specific processes that can affect how the results are distributed within those boundaries. It is, however, a moot point as to whether stochasticity is a cause or a consequence of complexity. The latest versions of the Daisyworld model contain elements that are stochastic, such as random genetic drift in the colour of the daisies.

Nevertheless, Daisyworld clearly has its limitations as a representation of a real planetary ecosystem. It may demonstrate some principles but it is far from being a tool for management. I first encountered this problem when looking at data concerning inter-annual fluctuations in the breeding performance of seals and penguins on the island of South Georgia, which lies in the high latitudes of the South Atlantic. This island, besides being stunningly beautiful, is rich in wildlife principally because it lies at a crossroads between different oceanic regions: the Southern Ocean under the influence of the Antarctic to the south, the temperate regions of the Atlantic to the north and the eastward flow through the Drake Passage around Cape Horn from the Pacific. Every few years penguins and seals experienced low breeding success. At worst, all the penguin chicks would die and perhaps 70% of the seal pups, involving

---

[1] *Reaction norms* are the magnitudes of reactions of an organism to a change in its circumstances; for example, the reaction of the growth rate of an organism to a change in temperature.

several hundred thousand animals. This was reminiscent of the effects of periodic El Niño events in the South Pacific but, in this case, there was no clear relationship to these events. However, using multivariate statistical analysis it was possible to get some idea of what was happening. El Niño carried some influence but so did variations in the pattern of distribution of the frozen ocean around Antarctica and the system of currents that brought most of the food for seals and penguins to the island. Although I knew that ultimately the breeding success of penguins and seals was driven by the amount of food that reached them during the breeding season, it was impossible to conclude what led to the occasional poor years because there was a complex set of factors that caused a reduction in food availability, some of which were also unknown to me. Moreover, I could not be sure if the factors, like El Niño, which I was looking at were independent of one another. For example, there is much debate about the role of Antarctic sea ice in El Niño variability. Processes like El Niño and sea ice were also removed by distances of hundreds to thousands of kilometres from the effect I was observing and there was relatively little clue to how such distant phenomena were connected to the seals and penguins, except obviously in some way through their access to food. Others continue valiantly to study this system and to narrow down the factors controlling its behaviour but, as in the case of the problems of the endocrine control of reproduction, I had come up against the same, unyielding problem of complexity.

In this case, the best that could be achieved was a statistical model that used a number of environmental factors to help explain variation in the seal and penguin breeding success. Although to the purist this may be quite unsatisfactory compared to a full mechanistic model and explanation, the existence of a purely empirical relationship can help to develop a broad understanding of the system being studied without the need to know how one part connects to another. This is an entirely different approach to that of Daisyworld and it reflects the needs of society because it cannot wait until scientists have a working mechanistic model of a critical ecosystem. These contrasting approaches are illustrated in Figure 2.3.

The empirical modelling approach (Figure 2.3) is probably the most expedient way to deal with complexity. It reflects how biologists have dealt with intractable problems for some time and it is the natural way that we and other animals make decisions in our everyday lives. A specific example in the context of biology comes from the generalised scaling relationships for the metabolic rate of animals relative to their body mass (Kleiber 1961). All the theory based upon surface area relationships suggests that metabolic rate should scale to mass raised to the power of 0.66. However, measurement shows that it is raised to the power of 0.75. Since the empirical relationship was first described nobody has provided a totally convincing explanation, although interestingly the latest suggestions (Garlaschelli et al. 2003) are gravitating towards the involvement of fractal structures, which are closely allied in mathematical

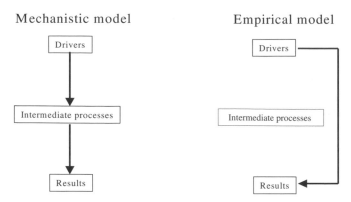

Figure 2.3. Representation of the differences between mechanistic and empirical approaches to modelling processes. The mechanistic approach demands knowledge of intermediate processes whereas the empirical approach, while accepting that these exist, makes no explicit attempt to understand how the drivers connect to the results.

terms to the *self-organised criticality* which is so much a part of complexity. In a sense, it has taken the biology community over 50 years to understand that this is a problem that cannot be understood by using mechanistic explanations.

The illustration of purely empirical solutions can be taken further in the context of animals' behaviour. There is a substantial body of theory and experimental study underlying how animals make decisions in the real world. We know that they do not understand their world, but they have enough knowledge of it to be able to make appropriate decisions based on simple sets of rules. An example of such a rule would be 'leave a patch of food to search for a new patch if your rate of food intake has declined below the long-term average'. Put another way, an animal will move on to look for another patch when, based on its recent experience, it feels it could improve its food intake by doing so. Even this rule may seem quite complex but experiments have shown that animals are fairly good at following the rule. The consequences of following this rule as opposed to other possible rules are that the animal tends to maximise its rate of food intake over other competitors. Through natural selection, those individuals that follow the rule tend to survive better, produce more offspring and pass on the rule-following behaviour to future generations. Some of the studies I have done on seals at South Georgia showed that they tend to follow these types of rules. Consequently, they have evolved a system for dealing with complexity which is purely empirical and ignores the need for any understanding of the complex set of interactions that affects the amount of food available. In fact, one of the insights I gained from these animals is that their poor reproductive performance in some years (referred to above) is likely to be the result of another rule, which dictates that they will defend their own survival against that of their offspring if food availability (measured by the long-term averaging rule) drops below a predetermined level.

SYSTEM PROPERTIES AND CONSTRAINTS

Ecosystems, like model complex systems, have components that do not behave in predictable ways. This reduces our capacity to manipulate different parts of systems to maintain a particular component in a desirable state. Much of the doctrine of *sustainability* is built upon the premise that we can manage our activities to maintain the state of desirable products from natural systems. The study of complexity suggests that this is likely to be impractical in the long term. Perturbations in some distant components of the system resulting from completely natural processes could result in shifts in the state of desirable products. Often we will not recognise the reasons for such a shift and we will take corrective action by adjusting our behaviour, such as the exploitation rate, in order to try to return the product back to its original state. Sometimes this could work but more often it is likely simply to result in an increasingly incomprehensible set of responses from different components of the system.

Nevertheless, the system itself may retain certain properties. An ecosystem may retain the same general level of energy input and biological productivity, it may retain the same number of species and it may retain a structure that conforms to a particular pattern. All this may endow the ecosystem with a certain degree of elasticity. This refers to the tendency for the ecosystem to return to its former state. One could easily imagine that ecosystems would be highly unstable if they had no elasticity because even the smallest change in structure could have wide-ranging consequences with wide-ranging species extinctions. This clearly does not occur.

The factors that give ecosystems their elasticities are far from clear. There is a debate about whether there is a relationship between ecosystem complexity and stability, which mainly revolves around forest ecosystems, but there is no definite conclusion about whether greater complexity leads to greater stability. It seems to me to be unlikely that complexity in itself is likely to result in greater stability because one can produce models with high levels of complexity but very low stability. There appear to be other properties about ecosystems that encourage stability and I feel that some of these properties are reasonably obvious.

If we contrast some of the most highly static ecosystems with the most dynamic then we can begin to understand the properties that might lead to differing levels of stability. Forest ecosystems are classically at the static end of the spectrum, with individual organisms of large size that live for centuries to millennia and which account for the greatest proportion of the biomass in the system. These ecosystems also tend to be internally highly spatially structured from the canopy to the forest floor, and this high diversity of habitat is probably what leads to them holding relatively large numbers of different species.

At the opposite end of the spectrum are pelagic marine ecosystems, which are populated mainly by small planktonic species or shoaling fish. Although there is spatial structure in these ecosystems, the structure is highly dynamic, with changes occurring on time scales of hours to days and space scales of kilometres to tens of kilometres, rather than years to decades within the forest ecosystem, and space scales of metres to tens of metres. In the forest, energy may be sequestered within the ecosystem for centuries but in the pelagic ecosystem it is most likely to be turned over in less than a year.

Pelagic and forest ecosystems also contrast in their relative stability, as measured by their tendency to return to their original state when perturbed. Both types of ecosystem have been the subject of massive levels of human exploitation. Whereas, in general, the sustainable management of forests is achievable (although political and economic pressures do not always allow management in a sustainable way), sustainable management of pelagic marine ecosystems does not currently appear to be possible. This is because the natural variability in the system is greater than the signal caused by perturbation due to exploitation by man. If left alone, forests will tend to return towards their original state (known in classical ecology as *succession*) whereas pelagic ecosystems will not tend to do so, partly because the original state was itself likely to be transient.

The drivers for these differences appear mainly to be the stability of the physical substrate. It follows that there is selection for species with life histories that are optimised to achieve greatest success for individuals, in terms of their genetic fitness, within the physical characteristics of each system. This is the key to understanding the complexity of ecosystems; it would be intriguing to know if the characteristics of different species will evolve to lead to a system with the highest level of elasticity that can exist given the physical limitations of the environment.

Therefore, where ecosystems are concerned, there may be hope that there is a limited range of structures that produce the highest levels of ecosystem stability in the circumstances. Some studies of estuarine ecosystems suggest this may be the case (Brose et al. 2004), showing that there may be a scaling factor for the number of interactions in an ecosystem and the number of species. Consequently, while ecosystems may appear at first to be examples of complex systems with unconstrained behaviour that is impossible to predict, we are beginning to see them as possibly being constrained by a set of scaling laws. Such laws may be the only ones that can result in ecosystems that have a long-term future. In other words, a process of natural selection may have taken place in which those ecosystem solutions that are inherently unstable have not survived (Fowler & Hobbs 2003).

The good news from this is that the management of ecosystems for sustainability may be practical so long as we understand the scaling processes that lead to ecosystem structures. However, we will probably have to accept that there is little hope of managing small individual components of an ecosystem in isolation. Instead, management of ecosystems will need to be more holistic, valuing economic productivity in terms of the way the whole ecosystem contributes to societal needs (and ensuring that societal needs are adjusted to what the ecosystem can be reasonably expected to yield) rather than simply trying to maximise the value of one particular component or group of components.

CONCLUSIONS

Complex systems rule our lives. In addition to ecosystems, which have been the main focus of this chapter, different types of complex systems include those from the business world, management/governance, economics and medical science. Our future well-being will depend on our ability to understand and manage these complex systems. In particular, continued long-term economic growth can only be sustained through increased use of natural resources or by increasing the efficiency with which resources are used. We know that natural resources are finite but an important route to greater efficiency is through better knowledge and management of complexity. Increasing efficiency often comes through increasing the complexity of the production and delivery systems within economies but, as we have seen, complex systems can have unpredictable outcomes.

Achieving sustainable economies may only be possible by learning from the way in which naturally occurring complex systems, such as ecosystems, are structured. These types of systems are likely to have been selected for internal organisations that are both efficient and stable. To achieve this, science may have to refocus its attention towards a more empirical approach to the behaviour of systems, including individuals, and spend less energy attempting to understand the underlying rationale for different behavioural responses to known stimuli. The intriguing feature of complexity science is that similar solutions may apply to the structure and management at widely varying scales. In other words, solutions to the management of complexity in medical science may have equal application to problems involving complexity at the scales of whole economies or ecosystems.

The title of this chapter was formed as a question and it is appropriate in these closing remarks to try to provide an answer. Complexity is proving to be an enormous challenge. From my own perspective, the mere recognition of complexity as a valid problem is a revelation and casts some light upon a large number of the unsolved problems I have had to deal with in research science. However, recognition of the existence of complexity is just the start. Traditional, reductionist science has probably approached its limits in some important fields. Complexity allows us to view systems as fractal structures where it is possible to describe the system in increasingly fine detail, as has been the tradition among reductionists but with a self-similar or scale-independent structure. Except in the most simple cases it is impossible to know all the detail about a system and, therefore, it is impossible to reconstruct how the system will respond to external pressures. Scientists are left making educated guesses about what components of a system are worth measuring because small changes in an unknown and unmeasured component of the system could have catastrophic consequences for the system as a whole. Science has certainly not reached its limits but it may have to dispose of some traditional ideas in order to meet the challenge of complexity.

REFERENCES

Ackland, G. J., Clark, M. A., Lenton, T. M. (2003) Catastrophic desert formation in Daisyworld. *J. Theor. Biol.* **223**, 39–44.

Brose, U., Ostling, A., Harrison, K., Martinez, N. D. (2004) Unified spatial scaling of species and their trophic interactions. *Nature* **428**, 167–171.

Ellis, G. F. R. (2005) Physics, complexity and causality. *Nature* **435**, 743.

Fowler, C. W., Hobbs, L. (2003) Is humanity sustainable? *Proc. R. Soc. B* **270**, 2579–2583.

Garlaschelli, D., Caldarelli, G., Pietronero, L. (2003) Universal scaling relations in food webs. *Nature* **423**, 166–168.

Hilborn, R., Mangel, M. (1997) *The Ecological Detective: Confronting Models with Data*. Princeton University Press, Princeton, NJ.

Kleiber, M. (1961) *The Fire of Life: An Introduction to Animal Energetics*. John Wiley & Sons, New York.

Lovelock, J. E. (1992) A numerical model for biodiversity. *Phil. Trans. R. Soc. Lond. Ser. B.* **357**, 383–391.

3 A Sustainable Environment? The 'Lopsided View' of an Environmental Geochemist

ANDREW S. HURSTHOUSE

School of Engineering and Science, University of Paisley, UK

INTRODUCTION AND PERSPECTIVE

Much of the research supporting sustainable development addresses the headline indicators of environmental quality and increasingly identifies the complexity of indicators and their relevance across global systems. A drive to identify the most suitable indicators is the focus of much research activity. Progress in this area in turn allows more effective management practice at the local level, often contributing directly to long-term regional planning. However, this process has often recognised the need to engage governmental, regulatory, community and business groups, in both dialogue and action, to deliver a sustainable future. While examples of 'good practice' are abundant, it is clear that environmental management, on all scales, can benefit from improvements to the relationship between the various sectors of the community. So where can the environmental research community improve our capability to assess and plan for a more sustainable future?

This contribution offers a view of our approach to understanding environmental systems and also how best to assess and manage the impacts of human activities on the earth. We have been developing this understanding for many decades, but still have a high degree of uncertainty about the description we have for the total Earth system. The fundamental driving forces are that human activities on the surface of the planet interact with natural components of the planet, often disrupting natural material and energy flows. This in turn presents a considerable challenge for environmental science to define the nature and magnitude of the impact and the flux of the perturbation, particularly in terms of historical and future direction and trend. For a future that allows human activity to sustain its progress while preserving resources requires a better understanding of the linkages between resource use and the development of society, and in doing so the need to cross traditional

Interdisciplinary Research: Diverse Approaches in Science, Technology, Health and Society.
Edited by J. Atkinson and M. Crowe.
Copyright © 2006 by John Wiley & Sons, Ltd.

disciplinary boundaries, which in turn requires new research skills and application.

Relationships between business, society in general and the environment are becoming increasingly important to evaluate. Managing the information produced or needed requires spatial awareness and understanding and the tools to enable that, as ultimately decisions made by or for the development of society or groups within it need to be as effective and sustainable as we can achieve.

The discussion here is based on the perspective from one discipline describing the chemistry of environmental systems. It illustrates how this approach can offer a useful perspective on the wider activities of society, introducing new concepts and potential tools to enable sustainable decision making and fully recognising the intellectual contributions from a wide academic base.

MONITORING METHODS: THE ENVIRONMENTAL GEOCHEMISTRY APPROACH

The Earth is essentially a closed system – except for energy exchange and the relatively minor material exchange through meteorite impacts and space travel. We have available to us a fixed inventory of material – the total sum of chemical elements, which are distributed very unevenly throughout the system. This distribution provides for great diversity in physical properties of the earth. As we move from the centre outwards we find solid and liquid phases in the core, a solid mantle and crust. The outer 'skin' interacts with the deeper Earth through material exchange through plate tectonic motion and outgassing as the solid Earth cools – essentially a large convection system. Interacting within the crust are the liquid and gas phases of the hydrosphere and atmosphere. The gas phase is the final casing, enclosing the Earth system. It is within these outer layers of the Earth that biological activity resides, with a complex and dynamic interaction between liquids, solids and gases, with very different chemical properties too.

The geochemist comes from a scientific discipline that has its origins at the interface between geology and chemistry. The subject has a long history but developed more rapidly in the early to mid-twentieth century as chemical measurements allowed the scientific community to collect increasingly detailed data about the chemical composition of the various parts of our planet (Krauskopf & Bird 1995). The ultimate aim of the discipline is to provide a chemical description of the Earth and its various components and attempt to understand the underlying scientific driving forces responsible for the chemical composition being observed. But more importantly, it is the changes in and to that composition with time – fluxes of elements and chemical compounds from one part to another – that we need to fully appreciate. These are important and fundamental questions about the Earth system, and geochemists have made major contributions to our knowledge of whole Earth processes. Geochemistry encompasses all the laws of chemical thermodynamics and basic properties of the elements and compounds, and has become increasingly quantitative, as knowledge of the chemical composition of the components is elucidated and material transfer links between these components (or reservoirs) are identified. One way of visualising the situation would be to envisage a chemical manufacturing site, comprising a series of sequential synthesis and reaction vessels, each dependent on input and output from the other. This is essentially the 'chemical engineering' of the planet, in which the process flow chart relates to the path of any element or compound through the system (see Raiswell et al. 1980 for a more detailed approach). The basic geochemical model is summarised in Figure 3.1. It describes the convection system from the perspective of material transfer between parts of the environment. The arrows represent transport processes and the ellipses represent 'measurable' amounts of material. Our detailed knowledge of the volumes/masses (reservoirs) and flows (flux) varies considerably from compartment to compartment.

As with any subject, the geochemical community has its own sub-disciplines: whether exploring for ore deposits as an exploration geochemist or

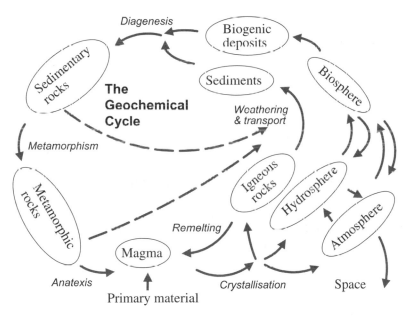

Figure 3.1. The basic geochemical cycle of Earth system processes. The diagram summarises major components of the planet and indicates processes responsible for transfer between the compartments. Our understanding of the composition and dynamics of processes involved varies in detail and with scale. For each of the chemical elements and compounds, the precise pathway through the cycle will vary (Adapted from Walther 2005).

understanding the formation of fossil fuel resources in the deep Earth as an organic geochemist, all areas rely on the generation of chemical data. The environmental geochemist focuses on the chemical processes that take place where humans have influenced the environment; in particular, concentrating on natural and anthropogenic environmental contaminants and their implications for human health and the environment. This includes impacts on soils, groundwater, freshwater, the oceans and the atmosphere and includes metals, non-metals, organic substances, nutrients etc. In particular the issues of risk, toxicity and exposure assessment are considered in terms of contaminant fate and transport, remediation and disposal, and source identification. The subject is obviously of great importance and support for the key issues we deal with concerning the chemical quality of the environment – describing its current state, assessing standards and evaluating improvements. At the heart of this is chemical analysis of samples representative of the compartment of interest – ocean water, urban air, soil, plant material.

There are a number of fundamental challenges for the geochemistry community, which both limits the impact of our work yet stimulates further research. The various reservoirs, about which we require chemical information, vary greatly in form and scale, often compromising our ability to obtain representative samples. In addition, we sample at a fixed point in space and time, often with limited success. Consequently the data produced have a widely varying degree of uncertainty associated with them – they are snapshots of the results of the process influencing the reservoir.

Reliable long-term monitoring of the environment is yet to be achieved, in particular to assess the additional burden from human activities. This is more straightforward for man-made substances such as toxic organic micropollutants, but difficult for substances that are found naturally, for example atmospheric carbon dioxide. Collecting baseline data to allow human impacts to be evaluated is a challenge geochemists have been addressing since the birth of modern geochemistry.

Pioneering work by V. M. Goldschmidt, the father of geochemistry (see Hitchon 1988), during the early to mid-twentieth century attempted to collate estimates of abundances of the chemical elements. For example, chemical analysis of glacial till was used to define average continental crust, and the careful selection and analysis of meteorite minerals was used to develop total Earth abundance estimates (Walther 2005). This then drives two distinct responses: (i) the collection of more detailed and more comprehensive datasets of chemical abundance over longer period of time (Reimann & de Caritat 2005) and, more controversially, (ii) the acceptance of the limitation of the model and a focus on defining the likely uncertainty associated with the description.

It also determines that absolute concentration information has very little relevance for geochemical studies. Data should never be viewed in isolation, but relative to some common reference point/value, that assists in the evaluation of the significance of the observation. This topic is also of considerable debate within the geochemical community (Reimann et al. 2002).

IN PURSUIT OF IMPACT DATA: POTENTIALLY TOXIC ELEMENTS AND COMPOUNDS IN THE CLYDE ESTUARY

An example of the approach to environmental geochemistry is best demonstrated by our short paper on chromium behaviour in the intertidal zone of the Clyde estuary (Hursthouse et al. 2001), which has been followed up with a more detailed evaluation with additional data (Hursthouse et al. 2003). The Clyde estuary in Central Scotland represents a fascinating geochemical system.

Estuaries in general are important conduits for vast quantities of chemical material produced by the weathering of continents facilitated by the hydrological cycle. Biologically they are important breeding and feeding grounds, subject to daily and seasonal changes, and the focus of complex chemical reactions as acidic river water mixes with highly saline, neutral seawater (Berner & Berner 1996).

Human activities also tend to focus in these regions, where communications and transport systems and urban centres have developed over time. The Clyde in particular has a long history of human pressure, being at the heart of a diverse and intensive industrial and population activity, growing from the early industrial revolution of the nineteenth century. The legacy is a system that has seen the decline of industrial pressures and associated discharges of point source pollution, and while the overall pollution burden has reduced, more diffuse sources are now of concern.

Chromium is an element of great importance to human society. It is a key component of many steel products and has wide use as a pigment and in leather tanning. It is also an element with a mixed impact on living systems – in one form it is essential for glucose metabolism and in another it is highly toxic. Both forms are stable in surface environments. Chromium is naturally relatively enriched in the local geology, and in parts of urban Glasgow, highly concentrated waste deposits are distributed in pockets close to ground/surface water and interactions with fluctuating water flow have dispersed the soluble components of these waste materials (see the special issue of the international journal *Environmental Geochemistry and Health* – Farmer 2001).

Our studies addressed an evaluation of the distribution of the element across the estuary and within the sediments, and how the element might be released from a relatively stable part of the environment into the aquatic system, with further implications for living systems interacting with the environment (Hursthouse 2001). This requires the collection of appropriate samples (sediment profiles, pore water, individual biota of different species) and in order to do that modifications and refinement of methods for both

A model for Cr mobility?

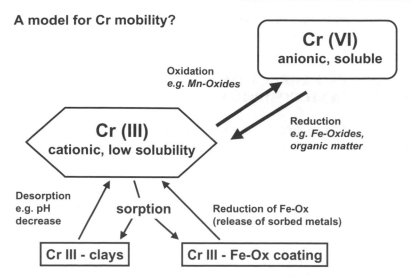

Figure 3.2. A summary of chromium interaction in soils, sediments and waters (*Source*: Whalley et al. 1999). Model used to explain processes responsible for observed concentrations of each chromium oxidation state.

sampling and analysis (Hursthouse et al. 1993; Morrow et al. 1997; Whalley et al. 1999). We also considered how wider impacts of pollution discharges influenced the local environment. A schematic process-based model of the behaviour of chromium in sediment systems, during our studies, is shown in a simplified manner in Figure 3.2. Again, the system-based approach describes the main reservoirs of interest (the oxidation state 'forms' of chromium) and the arrows the process steps responsible for change. Environmental observations made during our research address the content of the chromium 'reservoirs'.

The key to understanding the process is to ensure that sampling and subsequent analysis are of high quality – demonstrated by suitable quality control materials – and that relationships between samples can be clearly demonstrated. Collection of pore water, sediments and biota samples (sediment dwelling and filter feeding species from the local area) allowed us to test the potential for release and impact on food chain transfer through a very crude system model (Figures et al. 1997; Hursthouse et al. 2001). Results suggest that while environmental/geochemical factors do influence biological uptake (strength of sorption, composition of the samples), system baseline variability is an important consideration.

More important to these studies has been the combination of scientific skills. An understanding of the ecosystem relationships in addition to the source and behaviour of the target element allows the wider scope of chemical information to be understood. The collaboration between marine biology, environmental geochemistry and analytical chemistry enabled an appropriate range of samples to be collected for analysis using refined measurement tools, ensuring that reliable data were produced.

However, (eco)system variability often hides such relationships, particularly in the case of naturally occurring pollutants. The same approach has been used on more diverse and chemically complex contaminants – polychlorinated biphenyls (PCBs). These are toxic compounds found widely dispersed in industrialised zones and prone to bioaccumulation, particularly residing in fatty tissues in biota. The Clyde exhibits quite significant, but patchy, contamination hot spots, related to specific industrial activities (Edgar et al. 1999). By investigating the interaction of these compounds with site-specific properties, we have seen the impact of, for example, sediment particle size on the retention of the compounds (Edgar et al. 2003), which has important implications for wider risk assessment, with site characteristics having a bigger role on impact than basic chemical properties of the compounds.

TRANSLATING THE SYSTEMS APPROACH ELSEWHERE

The system approach used widely in the geochemists' approach to Earth process science easily maps on to those management systems that are used to regulate and respond to changing external drivers facing industry and the wider business community. These are not just in terms of emissions and pollution control, nor legislation, which is generally reactive and responds in a fragmented approach (NSCA 2001). The identification of links and transfer of materials and, importantly, information allows models of industrial operations to be constructed, which if comprehensive and refined enough allows the process to be more easily understood, and enables performance optimisation and sustained activity through an understanding of impacts and needs (Hursthouse 1996).

The approach being applied in this area is termed industrial ecology (Clift 2001), which can be defined as:

> the means by which humanity can deliberately and rationally approach and maintain a desirable carrying capacity, given continued economic, cultural and technological evolution. The concept requires that an industrial system be viewed not in isolation from its surrounding systems but in concert with them – the science of sustainability. (Graedel & Allenby 1995)

Implementation of this approach can be through a number of aspects of business/industrial operation (Clift 2001).

1. Materials basis:
   - choosing materials (design for recycle, improve processing)
   - designing the product (for reuse/recycle)

  – recovering material (physical/chemical properties for separation; recover
    value)
  – monitoring and sensing technology (tracking materials).
2. Institutional barriers:
  – market and informational (markets/exchanges; price/cost; scale)
  – business and financial (information flow)
  – regulatory (recovery/transport/storage)
  – legal (liability; favour innovation; procurement; trust).
3. Regional strategies and experiments:
  – Eco Parks; industrial networks.

Ultimately this gives rise to a new perspective on business and industrial
operations in which information systems and management are combined
with materials flux, and the management process takes a 'systems' approach/
overview. This is still a challenge and very few industrial sectors can demonstrate that this model can be achieved. An extremely good example of an
effective strategy from the industrial ecology perspective is shown in Figure
3.3. Here the basic steps involved in the production of polythene-based products (packaging, plastic components etc.) are shown as a flow chart with a
series of feedback loops. The main industrial and manufacturing processes are
identified from left to right, with processes required to return used plastic to
the system identified from top to bottom. The vertical operations require

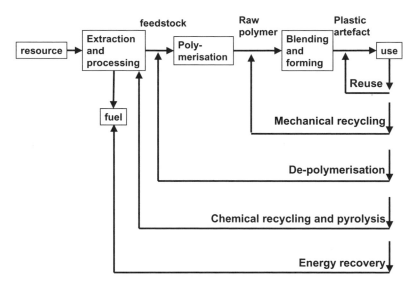

Figure 3.3. An industrial ecology for plastics (*Source*: Clift 2001). Industrial ecology
requires other external stimuli, such as legislation, economic viability of options or
alternatives.

increasing degrees of 'treatment' before material can be reintroduced to the process. By viewing the life cycle of plastic in this way, the design of the artefact can be considered to enhance reuse or other types of treatment, including the ease of separation/recycling as the artefact gets dispersed within society. This process system is relatively straightforward, requiring amounts and fluxes of material to be identified – the same observational tasks required for the geochemist to assess Earth system dynamics.

As a stimulus driving new avenues of research and seeking new tools to achieve the aim of industrial ecology, the approach has considerable merit and looks increasingly to become a driver of regulation and governance.

The idea of dematerialising industrial processes to focus on the service provided rather than the product allows cleaner technology to be adopted (Clift 2001). Converting commonly used products and processes into non-financial 'currency' can also provide a better understanding of net impacts. With each of the following examples successful conversion to the right currency with the right rate requires a full understanding of the system being described and calibration of common system properties with the alternative currency.

If you view the use of a standard motor car in terms of the amount of resource/material involved in its functioning, the impact of this widely used technology becomes much clearer. Results from a major resource assessment programme have recently been presented (Spangenberg et al. 2001):

- Average car = 1 t (materials input 20 t + 3 t catalyst)
- Function = max speed 190 km/h, range 500 km, transport 100 kg human being; 50% trips < 1 km; 80% urban travel, <15 km/h
- Accumulated use time of 3–6 months (0.5–1 h/trip).

It provides significant questions as to the efficiency of the technology in achieving transport goals (without including an assessment of other impacts). Further analysis of common activities is widely published. One example of interest is an assessment of the environmental impact of an international conference (Hischier & Hilty 2002). The various steps/activities involved in the conference were converted to emission functions for mass of CO_2 released. The individual activities vary widely, as seen in Table 3.1.

A key finding from the study was that 4% of the participants were responsible for 60% of the CO_2 emitted, due to their long-haul flight. A simulation of different models for the organisation of the conference concluded that in CO_2 currency, a virtual approach would be far less damaging in terms of greenhouse gases emission. However, they pointed out that the interpersonal interactions of a conference often produced far more significant environmental benefits through new academic collaborations and scientific discourse, difficult in a virtual environment! It is also a curious thought that in the academic system, the ultimate recognition of status is an international profile and invitations to travel to prestigious events – with, it would seem, in 'carbon currency', a more significant environmental impact.

Table 3.1. Analysis of component activities of an
international conference, presented in terms of kg of
CO_2 emitted (from Hischier & Hilty, 2002)

Step	CO_2 (kg)
Printed matter	1760.3
Cotton bag	202.4
Evaluation abstracts	478.7
Webmaster work	7.2
Secretary work	13.1
Travel activities	
By car	1066.3
By train	4049.3
By air – short	12334.9
By air – mid	14157.0
By air – long	43563.9

Clearly these case studies show that the systems analysis approach can offer new data, and new measurement processes. Different chemical currencies are perhaps of value where the element is subject to human intervention, e.g. in the case of fossil fuels. However, it demonstrates that ultimately human 'decision making', as would be expected, dominates the environmental impact agenda.

A SUSTAINABLE FUTURE? DEVELOPING TOOLS FOR (SUSTAINABLE) DECISION MAKING

A sustainable future for society clearly requires increasingly more diverse information describing the structure of society, its needs and impacts, and pathways to work towards visions of the future.

Currently we are involved in a project that attempts to bring a traditional scientific approach to study the quality of urban soil into the realm of decision making. URBSOIL (http://urbsoil.paisley.ac.uk) is a research network funded through the EU fifth framework, to evaluate urban soils as sources and sinks of pollution. Our new data is revealing very wide variation in quality across Europe and some interesting insights into soil science, in a manner very similar to our work on estuarine pollution. However, it is with the owners and managers of those soils that we need to engage, and to involve them in the investigation and interpretation of the results. How can that be achieved on an EU basis across many expertise, administrative and cultural boundaries?

The short answer is with difficulty, but the route to achieving this lies through the interactive use of information technology. Our approach uses the development of www-based geographical information systems (GIS) to provide visual results and associated scientific quality (Hossack et al. 2004). It gives us an opportunity to apply models of environmental processes to run through scenarios of potential impact. Environmental risk assessment is the end target for environmental quality assessment.

However, while data and data manipulations are relatively straightforward to undertake, the consequence of the results is less easy to assess. We see considerable value in the dissemination of that data and inclusion of wider opinion in its manipulation through consultation, reflection and feedback using the www. If we can apply transparent and efficient mechanisms to capture 'thought' and 'opinion' then this makes for more robust decision making. It also means that the knowledge used to make opinion can be captured in a 'knowledge base'. Techniques being developed and applied at the time of writing include computer-based 'Delphi' processes. This is a method where opinion is solicited anonymously, which forces, through controlled iteration, a group assessment to be made, highlighting agreement or divergence of opinion, the benefit being that decision making can be informed by all opinion and reasoning and is transparent in process and output. Perhaps not surprisingly, there are serious barriers to collaborative assessment processes, which have also been highlighted, within a diverse cultural and academic discipline arena.

These are potentially of major significance for the decision-making process, and to enhance collaborative and transparent evaluation of complex issues, the decision-making arena requires more careful consideration of their potential impact.

CONCLUDING OBSERVATIONS: A PAISLEY PERSPECTIVE

The University of Paisley has a rich tradition of research, crossing disciplinary boundaries and meeting the immediate needs of business, industry and society. More fundamental contributions to scientific research are embedded in its history and it is worth concluding this discussion with recognition of one of the institution's key individuals, Professor Lewis Fry Richardson FRS. As Principal of the institution between 1929 and 1940, he oversaw difficult financial times. It was, however, as a physicist and mathematician that he made significant contributions to the disciplines of meteorology and oceanography and fundamental principles in social sciences by developing numerical relationships to predict the likelihood of conflict. Details of these contributions are summarised and published in full elsewhere (Ashford 1985; Hood 1997), and show remarkable foresight in grasping some of the key issues in spatial data management and what we now recognise as geopolitics. He clearly worked with due regard for his own scientific discipline but saw where it might contribute outside traditional boundaries.

As a final postscript to this contribution, it is worth quoting some of Richardson's work, not from published scientific papers, but from the archive of lecture materials. The following excerpt is from Richardson's introduction to advanced optics:

You are on your way to become specialists in the mathematical–mechanical–physical–chemical view of nature. This view is very consistent with itself and it becomes more impressive the further we study it. As we climb the mountain of knowledge the landscape broadens. The whole universe appears constructed of electrons, protons and quanta. But allow me to remind you that it is only a special view. We have throughout excluded from your consideration all questions relating to living things. Thoughts, feelings and decisions, although we have and make them all day long, are not the subject of our studies here.

On the questions of artistic value, of right and wrong, of politics, of religion, we would remain, as far as merely scientists, profoundly ignorant. As these ideas are not our premises, so they are not our conclusions. Because we do not find them in our text books some scientists have felt them to be in some way 'unreal'. But this is manifestly an error.

The Arts men know better. The state of a man's mind is as much a fact as the state of his books. Admitting then that a physicist is a specialist who, like specialists in arts, has a lopsided view of life, we must remember that the community needs men who knowing thoroughly the intricacies of their special work, yet are modest and willing to learn about things in general.

A truly visionary statement that has become the guiding principle for much of the research agenda required if we are to achieve a sustainable future. Collaboration and contribution to research problem solving using a range of disciplines rather than one single approach can only lead to a more robust understanding of the system. But we do so in the situation where we must accept that any improvement in our understanding of the environmental system has to deal with transient observations, limited in scope and high in uncertainty, where borders are fuzzy.

This lopsided contribution I hope shows that transferring a perspective outside traditional boundaries offers new insights, with full recognition that the import of other perspectives can be equally beneficial.

ACKNOWLEDGEMENTS

I am grateful to a large number of former and current colleagues at Paisley, research students and research assistants and collaborators and funding bodies externally for their contributions to our research programme.

This contribution is dedicated to Sophie Hursthouse, who made 2003 a very good year.

REFERENCES

Ashford, O. M. (1985) *Prophet or Professor? The Life and Work of Lewis Fry Richardson*. Adam Hilger, Bristol.
Berner, E. K., Berner, R. A. (1996) *Global Environment, Water, Air and Geochemical Cycles*. Prentice Hall, Englewood Cliffs, NJ.

Clift, R. (2001) Clean technologies and industrial ecology. In R. M. Harrison (ed.) *Pollution: Causes, Effects and Control*, 4th edn (ch. 16). Royal Society of Chemistry, Cambridge.

Edgar, P. E., Davies, I. M., Hursthouse, A. S., Matthews, J. E. (1999) Biogeochemistry of PCBs in the Clyde: distribution and source evaluation. *Marine Pollution Bulletin* **38**, 486–496.

Edgar, P. E., Davies, I. M., Hursthouse, A. S., Matthews, J. E. (2003) An investigation of geochemical factors controlling the distribution of PCBs in intertidal sediments at a contamination hot spot, the Clyde Estuary, UK. *Applied Geochemistry* **18**, 327–338.

Farmer, J. G. (2001) Environmental chromium contamination – 18th SEGH meeting editorial. *Environmental Geochemistry and Health* **23**, 173–174.

Figures, J., Matthews, J. E., Hursthouse, A. S. (1997) Comparison of the influence of sediment and diet as sources of metals for diatoms and meiofauna. *Coastal Zone Topics* **3**, 66–79.

Graedel, T. E., Allenby, B. R. (1995) *Industrial Ecology*. Prentice Hall, Englewood Cliffs, NJ.

Hischier, R., Hilty, L. (2002) Environmental impacts of an international conference. *Environmental Impact Assessment and Review* **22**, 543–557.

Hitchon, B. (1988) Victor Moritz Goldschmidt: commemorative volume, editorial. *Applied Geochemistry* **3**, 359–421.

Hood, E. (1997) *Forward by Degrees – The University of Paisley 1897–1997.* University of Paisley, Paisley.

Hossack, I., Robertson, D., Tucker, P., Hursthouse, A., Fyfe, C. (2004) A GIS and web-based decision support tool for the management of urban soils. *Cybernetics and Systems* **35**, 499–509.

Hursthouse, A. S. (1996) The environmental impact of the chemical industry. In C. A. Heaton (ed.) *Introduction to Industrial Chemistry*, 3rd edn (ch. 9). Blackie, Glasgow.

Hursthouse, A. S. (2001) The relevance of speciation in the remediation of soils and sediments contaminated by metallic elements – an overview and examples from Central Scotland, UK. *Journal of Environmental Monitoring* **3**, 46–60.

Hursthouse, A. S., Iqbal, P., Denman, R. (1993) Sampling interstitial waters from intertidal sediments: an inexpensive device to overcome an expensive problem? *The Analyst (Lond.)* **118**, 1461–1462.

Hursthouse, A. S., Iqbal-Zahid, P., Figures, J., Mathews J., Vaughan, D. H., Davies, I. M. (2001) Chromium behaviour in intertidal sediments and pore waters, R. Clyde, UK (Proceedings of Special Conference on Chromium Contamination). *Environmental Geochemistry and Health* **23**, 253–259.

Hursthouse, A. S., Iqbal-Zahid, P., Figures, J., Mathews J., Vaughan, D. H., Davies, I. M. (2003) Chromium in intertidal sediments of the Clyde: potential for remobilisation and bioaccumulation. *Environmental Geochemistry and Health* **25**, 171–203.

Krauskopf, K. B., Bird, D. K. (1995) *Introduction to Geochemistry*, 3rd edn. McGraw Hill, New York.

Morrow, A., Wiltshire, G., Hursthouse, A. S. (1997) An improved method for the determination of Sb, As, Bi, Ge, Se, Te, by hydride generation ICP-AES: application to environmental samples. *Atomic Spectroscopy* **18**, 23–28.

NSCA (2001) Smarter Regulation: the report of the NSCA Commission on industrial regulation and sustainable development. National Society for Clean Air and Environmental Protection, Brighton.

Raiswell, R. W., Brimblecombe P., Dent, D. L., Liss P. J. (1980) *Environmental Chemistry*. Edward Arnold, London.

Reimann, C., de Caritat, P. (2005) Distinguishing between natural and anthropogenic sources for elements in the environment: regional geochemical surveys versus enrichment factors. *Science of the Total Environment* **337**, 91–107.

Reimann, C., Filzmoser, P., Garrett, R. G. (2002) Factor analysis applied to regional geochemical data: problems and possibilities. *Applied Geochemistry* **17**, 185–206.

Spangenberg, J. H., Femia, A., Hinterberger, F., Schütz, H. (2001) Material Flow-based Indicators in Environmental Reporting, Environmental Issues Series, no. 14. European Environment Agency, Copenhagen.

Walther, J. V. (2005) *Essentials of Geochemistry*. Jones & Bartlett, Sunbury MA.

Whalley, C. M., Rowlatt, S., Hursthouse, A. S., Iqbal-Zahid, P., Durant, R., Vaughan, D. H. (1999) Chromium speciation in natural waters draining contaminated land, Glasgow, UK. *Water, Air and Soil Pollution* **112**, 389–405.

4 Use and Abuse of Statisticians

MARIO HAIR

Statistics Consultancy Unit, University of Paisley, UK

INTRODUCTION

In a popular and populist book *Use and Abuse of Statistics*, first published in 1964 and since reprinted many times, W. J. Reichmann highlights the benefits of using statistics correctly as well as warning against the potential for misuse. This chapter takes the same approach to the use of statisticians in research projects and tries to explain the beneficial uses of a statistician within a research team as well as warning about the potential for misuse.

A major misuse of statisticians within research projects is that they are involved too late. In a mathematics dictionary, 'statistics' is defined as 'methods of obtaining and analysing quantitative data'; note it covers both collection *and* analysis of data. Yet many researchers do not begin to involve a statistician until they want to analyse the data they have collected. One student came to see me recently one *week* before her MSc dissertation was due with a large and garbled set of data she had collected over a number of months, expecting me to help her to analyse it. Every statistician could regale you with similar tales of people who come along with their 'research results' on reams of computer output and ask what they can do with it. Actually the best advice is usually to hang it on a nail next to the toilet, at least that way you get some use out of it. We don't tell them this because of modesty and the fact that we need the work. What we do tell them is please, next time, make sure you involve the statistician before you undertake the survey, not after.

Why should the statistician be involved at the start? Consider the word 'and' in the phrase 'collection and analysis of data'. The word can be used in two ways; it has a sequential meaning of 'and then' as in putting on shoes and socks; there is an order implied in this: a person would look pretty silly if they put the shoes on first. Moreover the two are independent; unless you are a real fashion guru the socks you put on will be largely unaffected by the shoes you choose. However, 'and' is also used in the parallel sense of 'with' as in coffee and cream. If you ordered that in a café you would be rather upset if they brought you the black coffee and half an hour later the cream. Most

Interdisciplinary Research: Diverse Approaches in Science, Technology, Health and Society.
Edited by J. Atkinson and M. Crowe.

researchers think that the 'collection and analysis of data' is like 'shoes and socks' when in fact it is more like 'coffee and cream'; the *two need to go together*. In the example of the MSc dissertation it was because the student had not thought about the analysis before she collected the data that she had collected so much data that was useless and not collected other data that was crucial.

If a statistician such as me is involved at the start of a research project, what can I bring to the research table? Generally my talent is in the method, not in the context. I cannot speak for other people but I have to confess that I am a kind of data slut; I will go with any piece of data that can show me a good time but I don't commit; after a few months I'm off on another adventure. I'm not picky either, I can work with health data one week, education the next, I don't care about context. I have worked into research of postnatal depression and back pain and I don't know the first thing about anything medical. I've worked on surveys of Heads of Schools and I don't know anything about education theory ('well, that much is obvious,' chorus my students). What I think I bring to the table is a way of looking at the problem, which is mostly back to front. I think about the problem with a view to what will happen when the data is analysed. For example, if I'm looking over a questionnaire I don't think in terms of the questions but in terms of the variables that they will produce.

One feature of analysing quantitative data is that generally you need to collect information about the same characteristics (variables) for all the people (cases) in the study. The result is a rectangular grid, like a spreadsheet. The important thing is that the variables must have the property of providing one unique code for every case, otherwise you cannot fill in the grid. Sometimes one question relates to one variable. For example, the question 'what is your age?' yields one variable 'age' with a unique code for each respondent. However, more often than not, one question produces a number of variables. For example, if you ask 'what are your three favourite television programmes?' then you need three variables to capture the responses. A consequence of the fact that most researchers think in terms of questions and not variables is that they often ask two questions in one. For example, I was asked to comment on a survey, one question of which asked 'Would you say that you are well informed about regional strategy documents such as the regional economic and social development programme or the regional operational plan?' I don't have any idea what these things are, but thinking about this question in terms of variables I immediately wondered whether someone could be well informed about the programme but not about the plan (or vice versa), in which case there were two variables here. However, if the programme and the plan were essentially the same thing then there was only one variable. At this point I asked the other researchers, who understood such matters, whether it was possible for someone to be well informed about only one of these. I wasn't asking about a theoretical possibility; if only one or two respondents might differ in their views to the programme and plan then it would not matter. However, if a substantial number of respondents did differentiate between programme and plan then there were two variables, and of course the researchers couldn't know from the response which variable the respondent was referring to. In fact it turned out that the programme and plan were different and that there should be two questions.

This example illustrates that my particular view of the research means that there are things I need to know and things that I don't need to know. I need to understand the logical structure of the data; I don't generally need to understand the grizzly detail. I regularly get involved with medical data and my helpful collaborators often provide me with papers to read about the medical condition and their treatments, sometimes with pictures. Most of this I can do without, thank you very much. One of the reasons I became a statistician was an aversion to blood and guts. All I really need to know is if the condition is good or bad and how it relates to other parameters: I don't need the pictures!

A statistician at the research table can also help structure the problem. Any moderately sized survey can yield a large number of variables. In a recent survey I conducted, a questionnaire of 30 questions yielded over 150 variables. That is a large enough total but 150 variables can produce 11 175 possible pairings. Hence there are 11 175 possible cross-tabulations or correlations of just two variables. Add to that the potential for interactions between three, four, five variables and the possibilities are vast – far too vast for any group of researchers to handle. All this from just 30 questions.

There is clearly a need for some structure. Researchers need to have some idea about what they are looking for and how they are going to measure it. They cannot just go and ask some questions and see what turns up. A colleague of mine is interested in the social and physical development of children, in particular whether a specific way of teaching them PE can boost their development. She collected a lot of data and then came to see me (whoops!). There was a mass of data. She had assessed social development by videoing children interacting in class and then painstakingly analysing the videos to measure each child for each of 12 minutes on 5 different aspects of social interaction such as cooperation and turn-taking – in all, 60 variables per child plus a few other demographic ones. Unfortunately, once the data was collected, she had absolutely no idea how to analyse it, no idea of how to get some overall measure of social development from the masses of data. The problem was the lack of comparability. A distinguishing feature of data analysis is that it is mostly done by comparison. The aim is to describe characteristics of a population and/or locate underlying causes by comparing cases to identify and measure how they vary on some characteristic. Unfortunately, simple comparison was not possible as the aspects of social interaction were heavily dependent on the task they were involved in. Some tasks involved turn-taking with other children, others involved turn-taking with adults while others didn't involve any turn-taking at all. Some analysis of the data will be possible but it will involve a sizeable loss of data and substantial manipulation of the rest.

This highlights another factor that most researchers miss, that often it takes a considerable amount of time and effort to get the data collected into a suitable format for analysis. If I quote that it will take me five days to analyse a set of data then at least three of those days will be devoted to cleaning the data and manipulating it into a format that is capable of being analysed. If you get a statistician involved during the data collection process, not only are you less likely to collect useless data but the time it takes to prepare it for analysis can be substantially reduced.

A research project that involves collecting quantitative data needs clear objectives. From these the researchers need to develop measurable variables often linked to some theoretical model of underlying processes. They need to think about this before collection of data. A basic problem with research is that the data collected has to be at a very specific and simple level; specific so it can be linked to specific variables, and simple to maximise the chance of getting a response from everybody. However, the objectives of the research are usually couched at a far higher level of generality and abstraction. The job of the researchers, especially the statistician, is to establish logical connections between these levels. De Vaus (2002) has termed the process one of *descending the ladder of abstraction* and it is by no means an easy or superficial task. But it is one that needs to be tackled early on in the research design – indeed, the earlier the better. The exemplar is a discussion of such a process.

The exemplar shows how the collection and analysis of data need to be considered together, and what a statistician can bring to the collection of survey data with an eye to how it will be analysed. However, it also shows that it is far better to collaborate with a statistician than consult with one. Collaboration is a two-way process, each party helping the other; consultation is a one-way process. Involving the statistician only at the end tends to lead to a consultant relationship: you are presenting a set of symptoms and looking for a cure. Collaboration is a far more productive relationship.

Collaboration is important for a number of reasons. A set of data can be like an old Gothic mansion house, full of beguiling nooks and crannies and secret passages. The statistician and the other researchers can help each other navigate a path out of the house without getting sidetracked. As I have said, I am generally not the subject expert but I often find that just by asking some fairly mundane questions I can help the subject experts reach a better understanding. A long time ago I used to be a consultant in a computing centre and as part of my duties had to help in program support. This meant that students could come along with any computer programming problem and I was supposed to help them. Actually I only knew a handful of programming languages and these were so old fashioned that they were never the whiz-bang languages that the students used. Nevertheless, I soon realised that if I just listened and asked the odd question and made sympathetic noises then, as often as not, the students would solve their own problems and miraculously thank me profusely for my wise advice! I know a lot more about statistics than I ever did about computer programming but I find that the same technique works just as well now as it did then.

Collaboration means that I can stop others going down interesting but ultimately useless dead ends because I can see that the analysis will not be possible. They, on the other hand, can stop me going down equally interesting but ultimately useless statistical by-waters by pointing out that something is not possible or that the results aren't real. Let me give you a couple of examples of what my co-collaborators can do to help me.

Sometimes the data I would like collected from an analytical point of view cannot be collected. A registrar in neonatal care came to see me about trying to predict a serious condition, necrotising enterocolitis (NEC), that sometimes occurs among young babies. In particular she was concerned that a condition sometimes present at birth, absent or reversed end diastolic flow (END), may be closely linked with NEC. Unfortunately the data was flawed. She had only collected data about babies who had END; there was no control group. When I asked about this she said she was only interested in babies with this condition so hadn't bothered to collect data about other babies. Most statistical analysis eventually comes down to allocating variability in data to different sources; if there is no variability nothing can be done. Actually there were two variants of END, absent and reversed, and I was able to show that babies with one were more likely to have NEC.

The registrar felt that this was of some use, but END occurs prior to birth and whether it occurs or not is out of the registrar's hands. What she really wanted to know was what interventions she could do after birth to minimise the likelihood of NEC. So I built a model that split the variables into two types, those that presented at birth, like END and birth weight, over which she had no control, and a second set of variables like type and rate of feeds that she did have some control over. Note that this distinction was not a statistical one but a practical one based on the experience of the registrar and it only emerged after a fairly lengthy period of collaboration. However, another problem came to light. All the babies with NEC had been breast-fed. Did this mean that feeding with formula milk was less likely to lead to NEC? That's what the data seemed to suggest, but unfortunately it was a little more complicated than that. Almost all the babies had been breast-fed, only a few had received formula milk, and the decision over type of milk was not random. It was always the (relatively) healthiest babies that received formula milk. I pointed this out and suggested that, for a controlled experiment, it would have been better to randomly give half the babies breast milk and the other half formula milk. The registrar replied that ethically she could not do so. She is obliged to give each baby the best possible treatment and as it is currently assumed that breast milk is best for babies she felt compelled to advise that they receive breast milk if at all possible.

Sometimes when I analyse data I see things that really aren't there, effects that are not real, and I need the other researchers who understand the reality of the situation to put me right. Some years ago I worked with a health visitor on research into the incidence of postnatal depression. We were comparing assessment of postnatal depression by health visitors in two health board areas. In one area postnatal depression was assessed using subjective judgement; in the other area it was assessed using an objective scale. We were interested to see if there was a difference in the incidence of postnatal depression between the two areas. At first the results seemed staggering; when the objective scale was used the incidence of postnatal depression was 19.3% (almost twice the national rate); when the subjective assessment was used the incidence was 7.9%. This was an important and statistically significant finding; unfortunately it was also not true! When my colleague and I looked more closely at what was happening on the ground, we found that, contrary to the policies of the health boards, some health visitors in both areas were using the objective scale sometimes and the subjective judgements at other times. What these health visitors were doing was using the objective scale as a confirmatory tool only when they already suspected postnatal depression through subjective judgement. This made perfect practical sense: the objective scale involves both the health visitor and mother in a time-consuming exercise, and it makes sense only to use it when it is most likely to prove successful. However, it makes comparison of the efficacy of the objective and subjective assessment regimes impossible to measure. In fact, we tried to isolate those health visitors who consistently used only one type of assessment and compared them. The sample sizes fell dramatically, and while there was a slightly higher incidence using the objective scale, it was not statistically significant. Worse still, it was no longer a random sample as those health visitors who used the objective scale only as a confirmatory tool tended to be those who were busier and had larger caseloads. The moral here is that collaboration with those who understand the context helped me to interpret the results correctly and stopped me making a fool of myself.

The above examples show the importance of collaboration. My contention is that you get better research if there are a number of different views of the problem. A statistician provides a very useful additional viewpoint but it is not all embracing. Rather unusually, I recently undertook some research along with a number of other colleagues from my department. This wasn't particularly successful and part of the reason, I'm convinced, is that we approached the problem in too similar a way – we lacked diversity. Statisticians understand the need for diversity within data in order to analyse it; I would argue you also need diversity within the research team in order to properly understand and formulate the problem.

BACKGROUND TO THE KILBARCHAN SURVEY

The research I'm using as an exemplar came to me towards the end of 2000 when I was asked if I could help the Kilbarchan Guide association with a survey of leisure activities among local residents. I've chosen this for a few reasons. First, they came to see me right at the start of the process, which was unusual (but, as I've said, absolutely the right way to do things). Second, they had a fairly well developed set of ideas on what they wanted. Third, the field-work was done very well and the response rate was excellent. Finally, the analysis fitted well into the wider picture. So I think that it gives a reasonable picture of how to undertake good quality research.

Kilbarchan is a small village to the west of Glasgow. It's actually a strange place in that there are no main roads that pass through it so you could live in the surrounding area all your life and never venture into the village. It often seems to me that the world has somehow passed it by, and it is none the worse for this. It still has a strong sense of community; churches, voluntary groups, schools and youth groups are all well supported. The Guides have a long history in the village. They currently use a hut, built in 1959, for guiding activities; it also receives a limited amount of use from the wider community within Kilbarchan. At this point I have to confess I have no idea what guiding activities might be; clearly I was never in the Guides, but neither was I ever in the Boy Scouts or Boys' Brigade or any of that sort of organisation. I suppose I have a vague idea that guiding activities are kind of wholesome things but the point is that I don't need to know what they are in order to do my job.

The Guides wanted to replace the hut with a new sleek, modern building from which they could not only provide guiding activities but also increased leisure and educational facilities for the village. For this they needed money and decided to apply to the Lottery Community Fund for finance. As part of this bid they decided to undertake a consultation process to determine the existing leisure needs of the local community, whether those needs were met locally and the extent of latent demand that the new hall might address.

Two members of the project management team, Jean Andrew and Christine Erwin, came to see me. Both of them were experienced Guiders (that's why I don't need to know anything about guiding) and both were also eminently sensible and extremely affable women. They had with them an initial draft proposal, which is replicated below (Figure 4.1). This was actually very good, a cut above most of the stuff I get shown. But it still required an awful lot of work to turn it into the finished questionnaire, which is also replicated below (Figure 4.2). What follows is a description of the journey from one document to the other.

KILBARCHAN GUIDE ASSOCIATION

IN CONJUNCTION WITH PAISLEY UNIVERSITY

SURVEY OF LEISURE ACTIVITIES OF KILBARCHAN RESIDENTS

We are undertaking a feasibility study to establish the need for extended Guide premises with increased use by members of the community in Kilbarchan.

The current proposal is to build a new facility, which would include a main hall, a lesser hall, modern kitchen and toilet facilities along with ample storage and improved access for all users.

The building is being planned to a high specification encompassing high standards of security and safety both internally and externally. Ramped access and facilities for the less able will of course be provided.

We invite you to complete this survey, which will be collected by a member of our group within the next week.

1. Statistical census question

2. Please indicate on the list below which Guiding units any member of your household is a member of

   Rainbow Guides   Brownie Guides   Guides   Trefoil Guild

3. Please indicate on the list below which village groups anyone in your household participates in

   Beavers   Cubs   Scouts   Venture Scouts
   Anchor Boys   Junior Boys Brigade   Company Section   Boys Brigade

Kilbarchan Singers	Junior Choir	Drama Group	Men's Club
O.A.P.s Club	Pigeon Fanciers	Tenants Association	Wine Club
Country Dancing	Line Dancing	Children's Dance Classes	Aerobics
Badminton Club	Beekeepers Group	Bridge Club	Play Group
W.R.I.Toddlers Group	Habbies After School	Civic Society	General Society
Church Guild	Glasgow Uni Courses	Bowling	Other

4. Which of the following activities do members of your household participate in outwith Kilbarchan

Golf	Bowling	Fishing	Tennis
Model aeroplane flying	Swimming	Computing	Indoor bowls
Health and fitness	Darts/dominoes		

5. Please indicate the location of the activities in Question 4

| Johnstone | Lochwinnoch | Linwood | Bridge of Weir |
| Paisley | Kilmacolm | Glasgow | Other |

6. Please indicate how many sessions of leisure activities each member of your household takes part in each week.

Figure 4.1. The initial draft proposal

	Person 1	Person 2	Person 3	Person 4
1 Session				
2 Sessions				
3 Sessions				
4 Sessions				

7. Are you happy with your current venues? Y/N

If not, please indicate the problems below

| Location | Suitable Access | Storage | Suitable Facilities |
| Catering Facilities | Toilet Facilities | Other |

Would you benefit from facilities for the disabled? Y/N

8. Please indicate which of the following areas would deter you from hiring/using the current Guide Hut

Kitchen Facilities	Toilets	Disabled Access
Disabled Facilities	Location	Cost
Lack of second hall	Hall too small	Hall too large

9. If any of the following were to be offered in our new premises, would any member of your household be interested in participating

Physiotherapy	Chiropody	Cardiac Renat classes/consultations	Alternative therapies
Optician	Sports Injury Clinic	50+ fitness club
Yoga	Aerobics	Slimming club	Other

10. Please indicate if any of your household would be interested in any of the following in a new Guide Hall in Kilbarchan

Music Appreciation	Floral Art	Cookery Classes	Sugar Craft Classes
Writers Group	Indoor Bowling	Senior Citizens Lunch Club
Handcraft Classes	Historical Society	Computing Classes Adult/children
Drama Classes–children	Camera Club	Language Classes Adult/children
Horticulture Club	Angling Club	Art Classes Adult/children
Pre-school breakfast club	Other

11. If our new premises were to comprise a large hall, a smaller hall, with equipped kitchen with catering facilities, modern toilet facilities, disabled access and facilities, please indicate on the scale below, how likely you and your household would be to use these premises for leisure and social activities.

Likely				Unlikely
1	2	3	4	5

Figure 4.1. *Continued*

KILBARCHAN GUIDE ASSOCIATION
IN CONJUNCTION WITH PAISLEY UNIVERSITY
SURVEY OF LEISURE ACTIVITIES OF KILBARCHAN RESIDENTS

We are undertaking a survey to establish the need for extended Guide premises in Kilbarchan with the potential for increased use by members of the community.

First, we would like to ask you some questions about the number of people in your family and the groups or leisure activities that your family participate in. This is to help us assess the level of demand for such activities.

Q1 For each person in your family aged 15 or over please give their Sex (M/F) and tick their age band.

Sex	Age Band			
	15 to 24	25 to 44	45 to 64	65&over

Q2 For each child in your family aged under 15 please give their Sex (M/F) and age.

Sex	Age

Q3 Please indicate the number of people in your family that regularly participate in any of the following village groups within Kilbarchan.

	Number		Number		Number
Aerobics Class		Country Dancing		Pigeon Fanciers	
Anchor Boys		Cubs		Play Group	
Badminton Club		Drama Group		Rainbow Guides	
Beavers		Glasgow Uni Courses		Scouts	
Beekeepers Group		Guides		Tenants Association	
Bowling Club		Habbies After School		Toddlers Group	
Bridge Club		Junior Section BB		Trefoil Guild	
Brownie Guides		Junior Choir		Venture Scouts	
Children's Dance Classes		Kilbarchan Singers		Wine Club	
Church Choir		Line Dancing Class		W.R.I.	
Church Guild		Men's Club			
Company Section BB		OAP's Club			

Other (please specify)

If no one in your family participates in any village group please go to Q6.

Q4 Are you satisfied with the current venues other than the current Guide Hut within Kilbarchan for the village groups that you or your family participate in?

Yes → Please go to Q6
No

Q5 If you are not satisfied please indicate the problems below (tick all that apply).

Cost of hire	Unsuitable access	Unsuitable access for disabled
Unsuitable location	Unsuitable toilet facilities	Unsuitable toilet facilities for disabled
Unsuitable size	Unsuitable storage facilities	Unsuitable catering facilities
Lack of second hall		

Other (please specify)

Q6 How do you see the current Guide Hut to be unsatisfactory as a venue? (tick all that apply)

Cost of hire	Unsuitable access	Unsuitable access for disabled
Unsuitable location	Unsuitable toilet facilities	Unsuitable toilet facilities for disabled
Unsuitable size	Unsuitable storage facilities	Unsuitable catering facilities
Lack of second hall	Not unsatisfactory	

Other (please specify)

Q7 Please indicate the number of times in the last year that your family have used the following health related facilities outwith Kilbarchan. Please also indicate where you used the facilities.

	Number of visits				City / Town / Village
	None	1 to 6	7 to 12	Over	
Alternative Therapies					
Cardiac Rehabilitation					
Chiropody					
Optician					
Physiotherapy					
Speech Therapy					
Sports Injury Clinic					

Other (please specify)

Figure 4.2. The finished questionnaire

Q8 Please indicate the number of people in your family that regularly participate in any of the following activities out with Kilbarchan. Please also indicate where you participate in the activity.

Number — City / Town / Village

- Aerobics Club
- Angling Club
- Art Classes (adult)
- Art Classes (children)
- Camera Club
- Computing (adult)
- Computing (children)
- Cookery
- Drama Classes (children)
- Fitness Club (over 50's)
- Floral Art
- Handcraft Classes
- Historical Society
- Horticulture Club
- Indoor Bowling
- Language Class (adult)
- Language Class (children)
- Martial Arts Classes
- Music Appreciation
- Pre-school Breakfast Club
- Senior Citizen Lunch Club
- Slimming Club
- Sugar Craft Classes
- Yoga
- Writers Group

Other (please specify)

Now we want to find out about the prospective use of the new Guide premises. The new Guide premises will comprise a large hall, a smaller hall, an equipped kitchen with catering facilities and will have disabled access and toilets.

Q9 If any of the following health related facilities were offered in the new premises, please indicate any that your family might be interested in using (tick all that apply).

- Alternative Therapies
- Cardiac Rehabilitation
- Chiropody
- Optician
- Physiotherapy
- Speech Therapy
- Sports Injury Clinic

Other (please specify)

Q10 If any of the following activities were offered in the new premises please indicate the number of people in your family that might be interested in participating.

Number

- Aerobics Club
- Angling Club
- Art Classes (adult)
- Art Classes (children)
- Camera Club
- Computing (adult)
- Computing (children)
- Cookery Classes
- Drama Classes (children)
- Fitness Club (over 50's)
- Floral Art
- Handcraft Classes
- Historical Society
- Horticulture Club
- Indoor Bowling
- Language Class (adult)
- Language Class (children)
- Martial Arts Classes
- Music Appreciation
- Pre-school Breakfast Club
- Senior Citizen Lunch Club
- Slimming Club
- Sugar Craft Classes
- Yoga
- Writers Group

Other (please specify)

Q11 Please indicate, by circling a number on the scale below, the likelihood that anyone in your family would hire the new Guide premises for a private function (parties, meetings etc).

Very Unlikely	Unlikely	Neither Unlikely nor Likely	Likely	Very Likely
1	2	3	4	5

Thank you for taking the time to complete this questionnaire. If you would like to make any further comments on anything covered in the survey please use the space below (continue on a separate sheet if you wish)

Your replies are completely confidential but if you, or any organisation you are involved with, would like to be kept informed of the progress of the new Guide premises please leave a contact name and telephone number below.

Contact Name

Contact Tel No.

Figure 4.2 *Continued*

METHOD

As mentioned earlier, a statistician can help to *descend the ladder of abstraction* – the process of moving from the high level of generality and abstraction in which research proposals are usually couched to the specific and simple level that the data is usually collected. This is rarely a straightforward process and usually involves a number of iterations, so it is more a case of nipping up and down the ladder a number of times. It's like repairing the gutter: just as you're about to start you realise you've forgotten something so you have to go back down again.

Once you have your specific and simple questions you also need to ensure that you reduce the possibility of error in collecting the data. Classically there are four possible sources of error in sample surveys: sampling error, non-coverage, measurement error and non-response.

Sampling error and non-coverage both refer to the way the sample is selected. Non-coverage error is the rather esoteric one. It refers to the fact that sometimes there may be some members of the population who have no chance of being contacted and so cannot be included in the survey. Sampling error is the one most people are familiar with. It reflects the potential that, just by chance, the random sample may not accurately reflect the underlying population from which it is drawn. Sampling error is the one most researchers worry about and the one they regularly engage statisticians to evaluate. This is what the statistical tests are for, to determine whether the results found in the survey are 'significant'; that is, exist within the population as a whole.

However, sampling error is only one source of error and it seems wrong to spend so much time and effort on it when measurement error and non-response are, in fact, just as serious.

Measurement error refers to the potential discrepancy between what is asked and what is answered. Measurement error can occur because of problems in question wording, response formats or questionnaire design. Non-response error occurs mostly during the fieldwork stage of the survey and refers to the fact that some respondents do not answer any or all of the questions. Involving a statistician early means that these forms of error can be reduced as well.

The following is an illustration of how the method was applied in this example.

- First, descending the ladder of abstraction to ensure that the research objectives were all adequately covered.
- Second, reducing measurement error by rewording and re-ordering the questions.
- Third, reducing non-response by redesigning the questionnaire into a more palatable format.

ANALYSIS

DESCENDING THE LADDER OF ABSTRACTION

The Kilbarchan project had as its central objective: *a survey of the leisure activities of Kilbarchan residents*. From this Jean and Christine developed four slightly more specific research objectives:

1. Collect information on current leisure activities.
2. Collect views on the current premises.
3. Collect views on other halls.
4. Collect information on the potential demand for the new hall.

Each of these was further refined:

1. Collect information on current leisure activities:
   a. Which activities are catered for within the village?
   b. Which are catered for outwith the village?
   c. For those outwith the village where do they go?
   d. How much time do they spend on these activities?
2. Collect views on the current premises:
   a. Is there a problem with the current hall?
   b. If so, what problems are there with the current premises?
3. Collect views on other halls:
   a. Are there problems with the other halls?
   b. If so, what problems are there with these halls?
4. Collect information on the potential demand for the new hall:
   a. How much demand is there overall for the new hall?
   b. For what activities is there demand?
   c. How much demand is there for these activities?

Finally, Christine and Jean had to begin to operationalise these research questions into questions that could be asked in a questionnaire (see Figure 4.1). The links between the objectives and the questions in Figure 4.1 are fairly clear but Table 4.1 helps tease out some of the logical gaps.

Specifically, there is a problem with question 7, which sought to do too much, whereas there was no question linked with research objective 4c, quantifying the demand for specific activities.

The first two questions in Figure 4.1 do not have a direct link to the research questions. These are general demographic questions that enable the sample to be broken down by gender, age and so on. These would form some of the independent variables. Independent variables are very important in quantitative research. These are variables that are used to analyse the data by comparison, which, if you recall, is a key element of analysis in such research. In many instances the independent variables would be crucial and would form a central

Table 4.1. The links between the objectives and
the questions

Objective	Initial question
1a	Question 3
1b	Question 4
1c	Question 5
1d	Question 6
2a	Question 7
2b	Question 8
3a	Question 7
3b	Question 7
4a	Question 11
4b	Question 10
4c	?

element in the research questions; for example, in determining whether there are differences between males and females, between old and young and so on. In this particular case these demographic variables were less central, and at this stage neither Christine nor Jean really knew what they would be, hence the bland first question 'statistical census question'.

Another issue that needed to be addressed was the unit of analysis. Was it the individual, in which case we would need one questionnaire for every person in Kilbarchan, or was it the household, in which case there would be far fewer questionnaires but one person would need to answer for the whole household. This is termed proxy reporting and, in general, is not advised because of the potential for measurement error. However, in this case the information was neither sensitive nor subjective. It was fairly non-controversial factual data so that a household questionnaire would not cause too many problems, but, as we will see, would require some care in question phrasing.

REDUCING MEASUREMENT ERROR

As you can see from Figure 4.1, Christine and Jean had already done quite a lot of work before they came to see me, and while they may not have descended the ladder of abstraction in quite the way discussed above, they had nonetheless achieved a reasonable result. However, there were still consider-able problems with their formulation in terms of reducing measurement error.

The most serious problem was that there was no link between the leisure activity information collected in Questions 3 and 4 and the measure of time spent on these activities collected in Question 6. Respondents could select any number of groups and activities in Questions 3 and 4 and it would not be clear from the answer to Question 6 which activity was involved nor whether it related to one within Kilbarchan or not.

There was also a mismatch between the types of activities listed in the wish list for the new hall in Questions 9 and 10 and the current activities listed in Questions 3 and 4. In particular, the single category of 'health and fitness' in Question 4 is developed into 11 separate categories in Question 9. Even worse, there are a number of education categories in Question 10 which have no direct comparison in Questions 3 or 4. Bearing in mind that the underlying idea in survey analysis is always comparison, comparison and yet more comparison, it would be impossible to compare potential demand with current uptake unless the same categories were used in both cases.

In the first redraft of Figure 4.1, Questions 3 and 4 were turned into three separate questions, one on participation in regular groups within Kilbarchan, one on participation in regular groups outwith Kilbarchan and one on health-related activities outwith Kilbarchan. For each question the number participating and the number of hours of participation were asked, and for those activities outside the village respondents were prompted for the location.

However, doing this made the questionnaire far more complex and difficult to complete. There is also a distinction between groups that meet on a regular basis such as the Guides, and other activities, such as visits to the optician, which normally occur on a more sporadic, occasional basis. It seemed that while one could ask for number of hours per week for the first, it made less sense for the second type of activity. Finally, there was the added problem that could occur if two people from the same household took part in the same activity but for a different number of hours per week.

When things start to become messy, a good strategy is to go back up the ladder and ask why you are collecting the information in the first place. Did they really need number of hours of participation? For management of an existing facility such detail may be necessary but in this case they simply wanted an idea of the current levels of participation. Yes, actual hours would be nice, but they were not necessary. Besides, most groups met for a certain number of hours a week so that length of participation was not a key variable. Here we have an example of expediency winning out: cutting out the hours question meant that the questionnaire could become simpler, shorter and easier to answer. It is also an excellent example of the need for collaboration, for discussion, between the statistician and the other researchers.

In the final questionnaire (Figure 4.2) there are three questions that relate to current use of facilities. Question 3 relates to regular participation in village groups within Kilbarchan; only the number of people participating is asked, not the number of hours. Question 8 asks about regular participation outwith Kilbarchan; again, only the number of people and the location is asked. Finally Question 7 asks about occasional use of health-related facilities and does ask for level of demand but in terms of number of visits rather than hours, which would be easier for respondents to recall.

There is a potential problem with Question 8 because this is a household questionnaire. Two people from the same household could participate in the same activity but in two different locations. This can happen but does not happen very often. The decision researchers have to make is whether to alter the whole questionnaire in order to accommodate a few cases (so creating lots of location variables, most of which are redundant) or keep it simple and put up with the potential for under-recording. We decided to keep it simple. In fact when this situation did arise, respondents tended to simply write two different locations into the questionnaire. But the way the variables were defined within the computer only allowed for one location for each club in Question 8. The problem was less one of collecting the information than one of being unable to analyse it. One final point, the analysis of the location variables was eventually calculated on the basis of distance from Kilbarchan, using just three broad bands so that the problem of under-recording would only actually occur in the unlikely event of two members of the same household engaging in the same activity in two quite widely spaced locations. The point here is that in survey design it is permissible to cut corners for pragmatic reasons as long as researchers are fully aware of the consequences; which is not at all the same as cutting corners because you didn't realise that the problem existed!

In the final questionnaire the questions relating to demand for the new hall were written to be consistent with those for current use. So Question 9 mirrors Question 7 in terms of categories (but does not ask about number of visits nor location) and Question 10 mirrors Question 8 for regular activities. Similarly Questions 5 and 6, which compare the current Guide hut with other venues, list the same criteria in both questions. In both cases this means that comparative analysis is possible. There is no longer a specific question relating to objective 2a, 'is there a problem with the current hall?'. It was felt that the vast majority would agree that there was a problem so that this question would be largely redundant. Instead one of the response categories to Question 6 concerning the problems with the current hut catered for those few who thought it was satisfactory.

Most of the questions on the range of activities include an 'other' option to collect any weird and wonderful clubs and activities that we were unaware of. This is a common trick in questionnaire design but one that is often abused. Typically, badly prepared surveys often list a few categories that come to mind easily then blithely stick in the 'other' category to catch all the ones that they failed to think of. Beware, the provision of a catch-all 'other' category at the end of a checklist is no substitute for proper preparation. This is related to the way people recall events. Ticking an existing category requires a mode of recall called recognition (do you recognise this club as one you attend) whereas responding to the 'others' category requires 'cued recall', which is cognitively more difficult (it requires more thinking). In general, when answering surveys, people try to avoid thinking and are much more likely to respond to a club when it is explicitly listed than write the name in under the 'other' category. There are also issues of uncertainty about whether a club that is not listed is valid and so on. We included the 'other' category but really hoped that it would not be used very often because, if it was, it meant that we hadn't prepared the question properly. In fact Christine and Jean knew their village inside out, and almost every club and activity was listed, so the use of the 'other' category was minimal. Incidentally, you might spot one of the activities in Question 3 of Figure 4.1 is 'Habbies After School' and you might, like the proof-reader of this chapter, think it should be 'hobbies'. It isn't, it really is 'Habbies', although I can't actually tell you what the group is. Another example of what I need to know and what I don't.

The demographic questions (Question 1 and 2 in Figure 4.1) also caused some problems. Most of the literature on questionnaire design states that such questions are best left until the end as they may be construed as somewhat personal and so affect response rates. In the early drafts of the questionnaire, these were duly placed at the end. However, when the survey was piloted (piloting is the term used when the final draft version is tested on a small number of respondents), there were clear problems with having these questions at the end. A number of people were perplexed that, in a survey on behalf of the Guides, the early question on participation in local village groups failed to list any of the Guide groups at all! They felt that the question on participation in the Guides should come right at the start. In fact, in the finished version (Figure 4.2), there is no separate question on participation in any Guide-related groups. They are simply included in the general alphabetical list in Question 3. This illustrates the importance of piloting each and every survey. No matter how carefully you design the questionnaire, you will miss things (I suspect there is a basic law – Sod's survey law? – that states that every questionnaire will be flawed). I've been doing this sort of thing longer than most and I am still amazed at the number of things that a good pilot will show up. I always advise people to carry out a pilot, and I always do so myself but at the back of my mind a little voice (my vanity) says – 'I'm only doing this because I know I ought, there is nothing wrong with this survey, I'm good at this, I don't really need to pilot' – and every time I am proved wrong.

Christine and Jean had decided that, as well as wanting to know if there were any member of the family involved in the Guides, they would like to know how many people there were in each household and their age and sex. The questions on household composition also caused a problem but this did not come to light until after the fieldwork when the data began to be analysed. When Jean, Christine and I discussed how to collect the data on household data it was agreed that it would be easier and less prone to both measurement error and non-response if we simply asked for the broad age bands for adults. However, for children, it was decided to ask for their actual age. This was partly because we thought that children's ages would be less error-prone to collect but also because the Guides wanted to get an idea of how much of the potential market they were getting, their market share. There is nothing wrong with this but it meant that our definition of a child was rather peculiar. We only got the actual ages of children *under 15* because after 15 they could not join the

Guides. For all other purposes a child is defined at least up to the age of 16. It meant that when we analysed demand by household composition we could specify households with pre-school children and those with primary school children but not those with secondary school children because after the age of 14 we only had data in the broad category of 15–24. The lesson here is that unless there are pressing reasons otherwise, always collect data in as much detail as possible. All we had to do was amend Question 2 to include all children of school age and the analysis would have been fine. We would still have been able to calculate market share for the guides by ignoring those aged over 14. We could always have ignored data that had been collected; we couldn't use data that hadn't been collected!

The last question, number 11, remarkably survived almost intact between the initial draft and the final questionnaire although the question wording was simplified and the response categories were given labels.

REDUCING NON-RESPONSE

So far I've concentrated on the questions and response formats, on the wording of the questionnaire. But respondents gather meaning from all aspects of a questionnaire. The words are clearly important but so is the design, the graphical elements, what it looks like in terms of size, shape and shading. Together these aspects constitute the graphical language of the questionnaire.

Design features are part of the process of reducing non-response, motivating respondents to take part in the survey. Why does this matter? It is a sample survey after all; so why should it matter if some households don't respond? If we think that only half our respondents will reply why don't we simply send out twice as many questionnaires? The problem is bias. Those who don't respond are different from those that do, they have different views, different characteristics, different behaviours. Doubling the sample size just gets twice as many responses from those who will respond and none from those who won't. To avoid bias you need to turn those who don't want to respond, the refusers, into responders.

The key motivational element in design is consistency. In the finished questionnaire there are a number of consistent design features. The places where respondents are to write their answers are picked out in white while the questions, definitions and response categories are in the shaded part of the questionnaire. The questions themselves are depicted consistently, in the same type face and font size. Response categories are displayed consistently and are aligned below one another. All of this is to allow respondents to use top-down processing to quickly complete the survey. A person uses bottom-up processing when they encounter new material and have to read and process all the detail before comprehending the meaning. When they are familiar with the material they can use top-down processing; reading just sufficient to recognise the familiar pattern and thus comprehend meaning. Top-down processing requires less cognitive effort and so is the preferred option for the respondent, and the quicker we can get them to use it the easier the survey will appear to be.

Other design factors in this survey aimed at reducing non-response included making the questionnaire in a four page booklet format, allowing as much space as possible at the end for comments and promising some feedback on the progress of the new Guide premises. Finally, an important motivational factor in terms of promoting the benefits of responding was the covering letter that accompanied the questionnaire. The covering letter emphasised the legitimacy of the survey by mentioning the survey organiser and sponsor, the purpose of the survey, and gave a promise of confidentiality and a contact name, address and telephone number. It also tried to promote altruistic behaviour by emphasising the wider benefits to the community of taking part in the survey.

DISCUSSION

I've tried to show in this chapter the positive potential for involving a statistician right at the start of a piece of research. In the preceding sections I've shown how a reasonably good initial research draft required extensive collaborative work to turn it into a questionnaire that had some chance of meeting the sponsor's objectives, using questions that would minimise measurement error and including design aspects that would reduce non-response. We have seen that every question had to be revised, often more than once, before the questionnaire was ready to go out. None of this is earth shattering; it is mostly the consistent application of logic and common sense. It does, however, require attention to detail. Strange as it may seem, these commodities appear to be in short supply, which is why many surveys are so poor.

I chose to discuss this research because Christine and Jean had a fairly well thought out initial draft document and had included most of what they needed, albeit not in a very polished form. But things can be a lot worse than this. A lot of other quantitative research I've come across forgets to ask huge chunks of relevant questions and puts in other quite useless ones. Worse, it tries to achieve too much and so fails to achieve anything at all. In this survey we didn't try to calculate the latent demand in terms of man-hours, broken down by category etc. We could have tried to do this and got some numbers but they would have been based on far lower returns, would have certainly had a large element of bias because of non-response and so would have been quite meaningless. Instead we concentrated on showing that there was considerable latent demand but we didn't measure it. We didn't need to, we simply showed it existed and was extensive.

In the event the survey went quite well, the response rate was around 60% and, crucially, there did not seem to be any obvious bias. The questionnaires were easily input into a statistical package that could analyse them and the results showed that there was significant latent demand for the new hall. These results were fed into a comprehensive document outlining the project in detail: all in all, a model of its kind. Unfortunately, the Guides were unsuccessful in their bid for Lottery funding as they failed to 'show sufficient disadvantage' (Kilbarchan is just an ordinary Scottish village). However, they did eventually manage to get sufficient funding from a variety of charitable sources.

And so it is that this story has a happy ending, as all good stories should. Early in 2005 I received an invitation to attend the official opening of the brand new Kilbarchan Guide Centre. I didn't go, but I do occasionally drive past and every time it gives me a warm glow to realise that my efforts have actually produced something real. When researchers talk about producing concrete results, they don't usually mean it quite as literally!

REFERENCES

De Vaus, D. A. (2002) *Surveys in Social Research*, 5th edn. Routledge, London.
Reichmann, W. J. (1964) *Use and Abuse of Statistics*. Penguin, Harmondsworth.

5 Research in Information Systems – Mine and My Colleagues'

ABEL USORO
School of Computing, University of Paisley, UK

INTRODUCTION

After reading the contributions of Neil Blain and Mario Hair my under-standing of what this book is about shifted towards what it originally was, i.e. writing *about* research and not a direct presentation *of* research, which my article on 'The place of ICT in global planning' is (Usoro 2002). So, I consider it necessary to precede my research article with a brief general discussion – written in a less formal style – of research in information systems. Apart from the conclusion at the end, the discussion can be split into: (1) where I come from (oh no, not geographically, though you may pick out that from my story, but research-wise) and (2) research in the information systems discipline. At the end of these two sections is an example of my research in information systems. A health warning: if you would rather go straight to what research in information is all about, please skip this first section. I hope that at the end of reading this essay, you will appreciate the multidisciplinary approach and method of carrying out research in information systems.

WHERE I COME FROM

It was not a structured journey to become an academic researcher. Born in August 1956 as the first son (second child) to a baker with a primary school certificate as the highest qualification and his wife with no certificates at all (but both keenly interested in education and cognitive exercise), there was much encouragement, sometimes even to the point of coercion, for me to do well in primary school. Apart from having to repeat my primary one, I was doing well; I remember taking the third position in primary three.[1] How did I

---

[1] In those days and where I hail from (I still have not told you), you had to take exams from primary one and failure at the third term would automatically mean a repeat. Yes, I did repeat my primary one.

Interdisciplinary Research: Diverse Approaches in Science, Technology, Health and Society.
Edited by J. Atkinson and M. Crowe.

feel about studies? I did not like it except handicraft and some arithmetic; thus you can understand my jubilation when in primary five, the head teacher ended his sad (to him, but not to me; at least I did not understand the full implication) speech to the whole school 'go in peace and not in pieces'. His speech was the last of the attempts to keep the school open at the outbreak of the Biafran war and the accompanying air raids in 1967. For two years, I enjoyed 'academic freedom' though being a half-starved refugee.

At the time I resumed school about 30 miles away from home (where war was still waging), the family had scattered and I was a child-servant to a master who very much enjoyed my skill at cooking beans. Unlike before the war, when I was fully equipped with school books in a metal box, all my benevolent master could provide was a big blank exercise book and a registration in a primary school which was miles away from home (passing other schools on the way) because he reckoned it was a better school than others around. I ended up in a 30% completed building that was used to extend the school facilities, which were overstretched by refugees like me. Though the teacher was very much feared not only because of his looks, with a 'Hitler' moustache,[2] but also because of his strong conviction in corporal punishment, I owe much of my academic interest to his strong dedication to education. At primary five, he introduced us to secondary school maths, including algebra, and surprisingly I could understand and enjoy what was going on in school, especially maths. I enjoyed the class for only a term before the war swept us a further 80 miles away, where I completed my primary six with distinction. Everybody insisted that my parents send me to a secondary school but they could not financially afford more than a one-year spell in what the government later considered 'a business centre that exploits kids'. The London RSA typing certificate I had just before the centre was closed down became my passport to economic sustenance and my introduction to an academic career which I did not foresee at that time. I read my secondary education by Rapid Results correspondence college (London) and with my credits I first went for a one-year professional teaching course at Cross River State University of Technology, where I came out with the overall best result (B1) in that batch. The certificate I had there combined with my other advanced certificates, including 140 words per minutes in Pitman Shorthand, equipped me to teach at the Management Development Centre in Calabar, Nigeria.

I went to the University of Calabar in 1979 to read sociology, psychology and social anthropology, then changed in my second year to management studies. My interests were so diverse that I kept changing – from accounting to human resource management (then termed 'personnel management') and then to banking and finance for my BSc Hons in 1983. I returned to the Centre to teach management and finance as well as to do a part-time MBA in stra-

---

[2] We kids did not (and did not need to) know Hitler's appearance to fear this man, whose name I have long forgotten.

tegic management at the University of Calabar. My first job in a university was in February 1988 as a lecturer in banking and finance but my curiosity about computing brought me to City University, London, in February of the same year, before which I did not use even an electric typewriter. Then, I attended South Bank University, where I worked like a hungry student to complete my PhD within 3 years in 1995.

My research experience started in my second year when in the sociology department of a university faculty of social sciences and I took the module 'Introduction to social anthropology and the study of African societies' (the module with the longest title I have ever taken). I enjoyed a brief ethnographical study of my village sororities. I was surprised how much I did not know until I interviewed the villagers. My BSc project on the impact of an agricultural development bank (NACB) on the Cross River State economy involved both qualitative and quantitative approaches. I used questionnaires and interviews, among others. The level of statistics was descriptive with chi square and not as sophisticated as the correlation and regression analyses that I used in my MBA thesis on the theme of organisational commitment (a misnomer, because it actually refers to the commitments of members to their organisation). My MSc at City University, apart from literature review, was more experimental and developmental in that I tried to build some computer software (middleware).[3] My PhD research returned to the quantitative and qualitative (in that order) approach of which I had experience in the past. I was studying the acceptance of computers by general practitioners in the UK. At the end of the research, I so much loathed my work (likely because I was burnt out) that I did not immediately get publications from it. Not that it was bad work, because years after, and to keep my promise, I sent a copy to a body that provided my major sampling frame. They took some months to send me a glowing commendation to my report. By this time I was up to my neck in full-time lecturing at Paisley University from 1996, and for 2 years did just that plus much administration.

At the end of the 2 years, I still could not bring myself to revisit my PhD report but launched into a new area, which resulted in my research example in this book. I first presented the findings at a business information technology world conference in South Africa, where an audience member made me feel my efforts were not worth while. Imagine how surprised I was to be invited by the *Journal of Global Information Management* to be among the few from that conference to publish (Usoro 2001). Next was a chapter in the book *Advanced Topics in Global Information Management* (Usoro 2002). That first major effort has introduced me to other IS research areas such as knowledge management, communities of practice, culture and virtual communities, which are some of the hot topics now (Sharratt & Usoro 2003, 2004; Usoro 2005).

---

[3] It was titled 'Network-relational mapping', which did not make sense to me initially when my supervisor and myself agreed on this title.

The new areas are not a departure but an extension of my major research area, i.e. global information systems.

When carrying out and reporting my research I tend to give priority to a positivist quantitative approach not only because of experience but also because of (perhaps) unconscious need for acceptance. However, key IS journals have within the past decade opened up to accept interpretative and qualitative studies and papers. I believe that a quantitative study should have some qualitative flavour.[4] I always begin with a theoretical paper, which inevitably uses a non-quantitative approach at the outset (cf. Usoro 2005). Among IS researchers, I am not unique in combining methodologies. You will likely agree with this statement after reading the next section.

INFORMATION SYSTEMS RESEARCH

Europe and America have played a major role in starting the information systems discipline and research. In Europe, and the UK in particular, we can point to the mid-1980s, when academics like David Avison and Guy Fitzgerald from the departments of computer science and management, respectively, pondered over the nature of information systems (IS), which at the time was in essence applied computing or data processing (DP).[5] By the mid-1960s, the scope of applied computing in organisations was expanded to management levels, and this introduced the concept of management information systems (MIS) (Davis 1999). In the 1980s and 1990s the merging of computing and communications technologies produced both internal and external networks of systems that linked businesses to both suppliers and customers. This development caused 'management' to be dropped from MIS. Moreover, computers are now applied not only to businesses and organisations but also to individual, leisure and home use. The term 'information system' seems to capture the current situation. Information systems grew out of computer science but are different from it. In their review of 10 years of the *Information Systems Journal*, Avison et al. (2001, pp. 3–4) paint a mental picture of a computer science researcher concentrating his attention on the computer which he stands facing. The information systems researcher stands in the same position but with his back to the computer, and faces people and the world that use and are being affected by innovation and changes in computer technology. I would adapt the illustration and say that in front of the information systems

---

[4] Birds of a feather flock together – my co-researchers and authors have also followed the same style. Sometimes, we complement ourselves. One paper is co-authored with a colleague who is more quantitative than myself and has no qualitative skills (Usoro & Kuofie 2006). I also co-authored, in 2003, a conference paper with a student who was more qualitative than myself (Grant & Usoro 2003).

[5] In the mid-1950s, computing technology started to be applied in organisations mainly for simple processing of records and producing of standard reports; hence the term DP or EDP (electronic data processing).

researcher is also the computer, since he does not ignore computer science in trying to figure out and study the interaction between computer systems on the one hand and humans and organisations on the other. The information systems researcher reckons that the outcome of technology application is not only efficiency but more significantly change that affects individuals and organisations.

In America, various efforts have promoted the birth and growth of information systems. Some of these were made at the University of Minnesota, which started its first IS academic programme in 1968 and became the first research centre in this field (Nolan & Wetherbe 1980).

On both continents, academics (and organisations) sensed the inadequacy of computer science (though very useful) in explaining computing systems and their human effects. The initial research focus was on tool and process design using engineering and generally hard science research approaches. Entity-relationship diagrams, structured chart and systems life-cycle models are examples of the output of these early researches. Since information systems and humans continue to change and innovate, emerging issues have been captured to form research themes. These issues expand the theoretical foundations and scope of IT to traverse the computer science discipline to applied psychology, economics, ergonomics, ethics, linguistics, mathematics, semiotics, sociology, systems thinking and even aspects of medicine[6] (Avison et al. 2001; Backhouse et al. 1991; Truex & Baskerville 1998).

The theoretical foundations and scope of IS are rich and multidisciplinary, as necessitated by the large range of multifaceted questions regarding the development, use and implications of applied computing and communication technologies in organisations, societies and individual lives. Examples of such issues are end-user computing, decision-support systems, and IT outsourcing, the last theme from about 1994 when it became the fashion to outsource (Claver et al. 2000, p. 185). More recently, e-business, e-governance, knowledge management, wireless and mobile systems, and global issues have emerged.

This polycentric nature of research issues in information systems attracts not only a cross-disciplinary approach but also multi-methodologies, which can broadly be classified into empirical and theoretical or non-empirical. Claver et al. (2000) divide theoretical studies into conceptual, illustrative and applied concepts. Empirical studies as classified by Van Horn (1973) and used by others (Hamilton & Ives 1982, pp. 61–77) are case studies, field studies, field experiments and laboratory experiments.

A theoretical researcher projects his ideas and speculations, which are not primarily based on systematic observation in the way that empirical studies are carried out. Conceptual studies propound frameworks, models or theories, along with their reasonings and explanations. Illustrative studies answer the

---

[6] Recently, new disciplines like medical informatics have emerged to address not only the applied computing aspects of handling medical records but also the human and organisational aspects of applying computing to the health sector.

questions 'what?' and 'how?' rather than 'why?' and therefore guide practice. They provide the recipe for carrying out action. Lastly, applied concepts stress both the conceptual and the illustrative.

Empirical studies seek to understand reality by gathering observable evidence. Observation using case studies is increasingly used in IS research though it is criticised for producing mostly anecdotal evidence and inadequate scientific rigour. With field study, several organisations are analysed in terms of one or a number of variables. To succeed, this kind of study requires a large amount of data to be collected, likely with the use of questionnaires. Nowadays, Internet questionnaires are popular. In 2004, I met an IS researcher who had set up large panels of Internet respondents. His university has now taken ownership of the system, which helps to get respondents for questionnaires, thus tackling the nagging problem of questionnaire non-response (http://istprojects.syr.edu/~studyresponse/studyresponse/index.htm).

Field experiment involves applying experimental design and control to organisational study such that there is a control group. Though they apparently promote scientific rigour, field experiments are rare in IS research because of the difficulty of controlling for variables in real-life situations. Laboratory experiments are more rarely used in IS research because the artificial situations created for this method of study may be too unrealistic to apply to real life, which IS is concerned with. Thus a survey of articles published within the decade beginning 1981 of two major IS journals (*Management Information Systems Quarterly* and *Information and Management*) revealed only a total of 7.5% of studies performed by this methodology (Claver et al. 2000, p. 187). The same survey showed that overall, empirical studies are the most popular (68.7%) as against theoretical studies (31.3%). A review of 157 articles published in *IS Journal* for the decade beginning 1991 revealed that 24 are predominantly case studies, 17 dependent on surveys or field studies, and 69 discursive (Avison et al. 2001, p. 6).

Leading IS journals such as *MIS* ten years ago would not accept a research or theory article if it were not based on a set of well-defined hypotheses, unbiased and reproducible evidence, often involving the collection of large quantities of statistical data. Nowadays, the scene has changed with *IS Journal* within the decade ending 2001 accepting papers based on case studies, action research, hermeneutics, critical thinking, agency theory, speech act theory, postmodernist theory, grounded theory, feminist theory, personal construct theory and phenomenological research (Avison et al. 2001, p. 14).

A subset of information systems researchers who have recently caught my attention is the critical information systems researchers. Their critical epistemology rejects the idea that objective science and technological advancement bring human progress. In the words of one critical systems researcher, 'its [critical epistemology's] point of departure is in the position that science and engineering, if practised as technical/rational activities, prevent us from addressing questions on the moral nature of techno-scientific knowledge and make us blind to the socio-political forces that are implicated in the formation of all knowledge claims' (Avgerou 2005, p. 107). Interestingly, Avgerou of the London School of Economics was responding to McGrath (2005), who was arguing for a more explicit methodological account of critical research in information systems. Avgerou expressed his suspicion that methodological emphasis tends to defend the philosophical underpinnings of the status quo which critical research seeks to vehemently question. There is the fear that sticking to much methodology may disenfranchise the voice of research performed on the unfortunate members of humanity who may be suffering the effects of orthodox information systems theories and practices. Walsham (2005, p. 112) also, in his defence of the relatively less explicit methodological account, sums up a critical stance as 'focused on what is wrong with the world rather than what is right. It tends to focus on issues such as asymmetries of power, alienation, disadvantaged groups or structural inequality'. It is therefore understandable why critical IS researchers often use interpretative and eclectic approaches.

CONCLUSION

The discipline of information systems emerged from computer science but is different from it. Information systems research themes can broadly be split into technological and human factors. It is realised that much system failure is caused more by the latter than the former (Avison et al. 2001, p. 5). Information systems research therefore does not shy away from employing any relevant reference discipline such as management, social science or engineering, to solve the complex and multifaceted challenges of innovation in computer technology and its impact on individuals and organisations. In so doing, both the theories and research methods of the reference disciplines have found ready use in investigating the workings and effects of information systems. As the field of computing and communications technologies as well as human society continues to change, information systems research will accordingly respond. This essay precedes a presentation of an empirical work I did in information systems.

ICT IN GLOBAL PLANNING: A THEORETICAL MODEL AND A PILOT STUDY

INTRODUCTION

Both researchers and practitioners unanimously agree to the increasing tendency for organisations to operate across national borders (Hull 1987; Hax 1989; Ohmae 1989; Ietto-Gillies 1997; *Business Week* 2000, p. 113; Grosse 2000, p. vii; Harvey et al. 2000). The crossing of national borders is traditionally termed 'internationalisation' (Taggart & McDermott 1993, p. 4) and can take different forms of engagement. At the lower end of the scale is indirect export whereby a company distributes its products abroad by using third parties (Toyne & Walters 1993, p. 114). At the highest level is globalisation, whereby there is no distinction between domestic and foreign operations but there is freedom to source or allocate resources or operations to, and choose markets from, any strategically advantageous location (Humes 1993; Ball & McCullock 1996). All international businesses, irrespective of their cross-border involvement, must constantly evaluate their positions to decide, first, whether to maintain their positions, or to move up or down the scale of internationalisation. Second, they have to decide *how* to maintain or change their positions. In these two respects, we can safely conclude that all international firms perform some form of global planning since international companies that may be termed 'non-global' have to constantly assess whether or not to globalise. Non-global international organisations are pressured by strong global, social, political and economic forces to develop global strategies (Humes 1993, p. 25; Govindarajan & Gupta 2000, pp. 5–10). Alongside these forces or drivers are advances in information and communication technologies (ICT) to bridge the geographical, time and knowledge distances experienced in global operations[7] (Uenohara 1992, p. 402; Campbell et al. 1999; Currie 2000).

The rest of this paper (a) explains briefly what is involved in global planning; (b) discusses the role of ICT in global planning; (c) identifies problems and justifies the need for investigation; (d) proposes a hypothetical model; (e) states the method of study; (f) presents and discusses the findings of a pilot study, including its major conclusions and recommendations; and (g) highlights areas for further research.

WHAT GLOBAL PLANNING IS

It is hard to find a clear definition of global planning in the literature but the concept is embedded in various contexts, for example, health care and the provision of public utilities (Ryan 1990, pp. 61–63; Yehia et al. 1995, p. 10). This research locates global planning in the context of strategic planning, which is the managerial act of setting long-term goals and objectives based on the strengths and weaknesses of the organisation, on the one hand, and the threats posed and opportunities offered by the environment, on the other (Ansoff 1979; Johnson & Scholes 1997; Wheelen 2000).

Strategic planning has been well grounded in literature since the Harvard Business School in the 1920s developed the Harvard Policy Model (Carter 1999, p. 1). However, its popularity fell in the 1980s due to the increased pace

---

[7] The International Monetary Fund (1997) defines 'globalisation' as 'the growing economic interdependencies of countries worldwide through the increasing volume and variety of cross-border transactions in goods and services and of international capital flows, and also through the rapid and widespread diffusion of technology' (p. 45).

of environmental changes that made obsolete and irrelevant most of the long-term planning done over a long period of time and by the few at the top of the organisational hierarchy. Consequently, total quality management (TQM), business process reengineering (BPR), value chain analyses and other new concepts emerged as short-term planning techniques to match the changing environments and capture customer preference. Besides, in organisations with a flatter structure, the idea of central planning and its top-down process became unpopular with middle managers, who were increasingly exposed to the environment and needed to respond rapidly without being tied to handed-down plans. Academics reasoned that rather than strategic planning, organisational learning, employee empowerment and agility are what contribute to competitive advantage. Feurer and Chaharbaghi (1995) give a comprehensive review of the history of strategy development, with the main theme that 'the dynamic environments of today require a more dynamic approach to strategy development' (p. 11).

Interestingly, strategic planning has recently re-emerged as the unifying organisational process that directs its different members towards optimal achievements (Carter 1999; Desai 2000; Quazi 2001). New research proves that strategic planning *does* contribute to competitive advantage. An example is one carried out by Desai (2000), which confirms that the explicit statement of companies about their strategic planning focus, function or orientation has an immediate positive effect on their share values. Instead of being viewed as a discouraging factor to strategic planning, the increasing uncertainty of the environment provides the impetus for managers to use the tools to cope with the complex, changing environments and to shape organisational responses (Morgan & Piercy 1993; Quazi 2001).

Global planning is strategic planning with emphasis on the need to take a worldview of the changing environments and to develop the ability to pull and pool together knowledge that may be spread across the globe. In contrast to traditional strategic planning, global planning is battered more by environmental changes and diversity; and planning needs to be simplified, speedy and flexible. In line with the current view of strategic planning, emphasis has to be placed on the process (the learning process) rather than the products (plans) themselves, which are snapshots and quickly become history (Carter 1999, p. 48). A large amount of information has to be easily and rapidly pulled together and analysed, and critical success factors quickly identified. Involvement of a greater number of organisational members is vital to both modern strategic planning and global planning. Planning has to be integrated with action[8] and there has to be readiness to change direction, when necessary (Feurer & Chaharbaghi 1995, p. 5; Chakravarthy & Lorange 1991).

---

[8] Hertzberg (1995) stated that 'every failure of implementation is, by definition, also a failure of formulation. The real blame [of unsuccessfully planned strategies] has to be laid, neither on formulation or on implementation, but on *the very separation of the two* . . . It is the disassociation of thinking from acting that lies closer to the root of the problem' (p. 285).

Global planning is influenced by global stance (ethnocentric, polycentric, regiocentric, geocentric or some mixture of these viewpoints), which is an aspect of an organisation's philosophy (Rugman & Hodgetts 1995, p. 215; Buckley 1998, p. 13; Holt 1998, p. 236). The considered decision to take a particular stance can also be viewed as an output of global planning at a high level. An ethnocentric stance places emphasis on the country of origin, for example, in personnel issues (Hill 1998, pp. 448–453). A polycentric view localises business in each global location, while a regiocentric position does the same for trade regions, e.g. the EU. The geocentric philosophy emphasises total globalisation or standardisation of goods, services and practices with little or no adaptation to local needs. A host of global, national and company factors should be taken into consideration to decide on and constantly review the philosophy in the light of rapidly changing global economic, political and cultural situations. Managers face a difficult balancing act between meeting the demands of the increasing global converged economy and the need to support national policies that provide distinctive competitive advantage (Doremus et al. 1999, p. 165).

New developments in ICT present global managers with the potential to perform these tasks more easily and faster (Alkhafaji 1991).

HOW ICT COULD HELP

Though ICT is not a replacement for human judgement and imagination, it can assist global planning in:

- quickly identifying internal strengths and weaknesses;
- performing environmental scanning;
- bridging the geographical distance between planners;
- simplifying the planning process.

The first stage of planning is to discover the internal resources and capabilities for they provide information on organisational strength (Penrose 1963; Kay 1993, pp. 17–37). For many organisations, this information may be distributed at many locations of the organisation as well as the world. Provided this information is in electronic form and the information systems are compatible, the information can be pulled together irrespective of distance. Internet technology along with developments in enterprise information systems (e.g. SAP) presents the potential for achieving these aims. Moreover, recent developments in the Internet communication language, termed XML, promise to make possible the exchange of more meaningful information. Thus, information can be classified, transferred, analysed and presented at greater speed. This capability can also be useful when performing environmental scanning.

According to Chae and Hill (1996, pp. 880–891) the most disruptive influences to global planning efforts tend to come from the environment. Thus, it is important for every organisation to identify and constantly monitor environmental factors relevant to its operations so as to take advantage of their opportunities and avoid or cope with their threats. A number of Internet-based technologies and applications have been developed to perform these tasks. Besides XML, Fletcher and Donaghy (1994, pp. 4–18), for instance, write about computer systems for monitoring competitors' moves.

The geographical spread of planners requires collaborative working technologies. Groupware technologies fall into this category. They provide electronic conferencing and enable users to share the same source of information and exchange ideas. Thus, Fulmer and Sashkin (1995, pp. 26–31) considered groupware also as an essential tool for global learning organisations, and Stough et al. (2000, pp. 370–378) described groupware as a supporting technology for communication, information storage and retrieval, and decision making in virtual teams.

Sokol's (1992) study indicated that simplifying the strategic planning process yielded benefits. These benefits include saving time in developing a plan and shortening the lead time to implement it, making the plan easier to understand, focusing better on only the most relevant business issues, and assembling a more consistent strategy for the whole company.

ICT has the potential of simplifying the planning process. For example, business and planning models such as SWOT, PEST and Porter's Value Chain and 5-point models can be built into ICT, thereby simplifying and quickening the processing of information (Rugman & Hodgetts 1995, pp. 218, 221–222). Moreover, using the presentation facilities of ICT, different perspectives of information can be displayed with the ability to easily switch between highly summarised and detailed views of information. ICT should facilitate knowledge sharing, which is needed for global planning. The simplification of the global planning process opens the opportunity for relatively small businesses to enter the global market with relative ease (Tetteh & Burn 2001).

PROBLEM

Reid's (1989) face-to-face study of 100 chief and senior executives in Scotland revealed that companies were failing to effectively utilise the creative talents of key people in the harnessing of information. Consequently, they were failing to gain valuable insights and to obtain essential collective interpretations of critical issues and events that affect their strategic planning process. Apparently, the situation has not significantly changed, especially in global planning, despite the potential that ICT offers to the planning process (Hagmann & McCahon 1993, pp. 183–192; Houben et al. 1999; Usoro 2001, pp. 17–24).

Moreover, no theoretical framework appears to exist for examining the use of ICT for global planning. Thus, Ho (1996) was able to state that 'the connection between strategy and IT has not been clearly articulated with respect to a finite set of concepts, analytical framework, and normative prescriptions' (p. 77). Such a framework is needed to attempt to understand the current use of ICT for global planning and also to provide guidance on how to improve the use of ICT in this area.

A HYPOTHETICAL MODEL: FACTORS THAT INFLUENCE THE USE OF ICT FOR GLOBAL PLANNING

The literature does not reveal an existing and well-researched theory that explains the use of ICT for global planning. Using a literature and experience survey, Usoro (2001, pp. 17–23; 2002, pp. 136–149) made an initial attempt at designing a model to explain and predict the use of ICT for global planning. He hypothesised that factors could be grouped under organisational, information technology, personal and infrastructural elements to form relationships as shown in Figure 5.1.

Organisational factors refer to profile items such as size, years in business and their stance along the ethnocentric and geocentric continuum (Özsomer et al. 1997). Jeannet (1999, p. 28) has described the stance as a 'global mindset' which determines the success of global planning. This research takes a step further by examining the effect of the mindset on the use of ICT in planning. The closer an organisation is to the ethnocentric end, the lower the level of globalisation, and the closer it is to the geocentric end, the higher would be the level of globalisation. Does the level of globalisation correlate positively with the use of global planning technologies? Another factor closely related to the level of globalisation is involvement in global planning. Do companies that are more involved in global planning tend to use information technology more? Other organisational factors of interest are years in business and

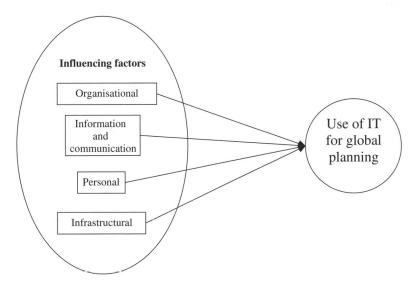

Figure 5.1. Hypothetical model of factors influencing the use of ICT in global planning.

number of countries in which a company operates. Do these make any difference with regard to the use of information technology for global planning?

ICT factors refer to the attributes of ICT itself. The mere presence of integrative and collaborative ICT does not guarantee a seamless and supportive working environment (Grant 2003, pp. 159–175). ICT's relevance and level of support to global planners are called into question. It should support group working as well as possess the following attributes of executive support systems (ESS) (Usoro 1998):

- easy user interface for learning and using the system;
- ability to easily switch between highly summarised and detailed views of information;
- on-demand link to internal information for indication of strengths and weaknesses;
- statistical analysis tool;
- ad hoc query and sensitivity analysis handling;
- access to external data pools – non-company data;
- flexibility to solve diverse problems;
- constant review of decisions, before and after implementation;
- report and presentation facilities;
- support for optimisation, satisficing and heuristic approaches;
- use and provision of accurate, understandable, complete and timely information.

Ives et al. (1993) have also pointed out the need for compatibility of systems when they state that 'few multinational firms can boast of . . . globally integrated information processing environment' (p. 114). Incompatible ICT systems present a barrier instead of helping global planning and it is one of the aims of emerging technologies such as the Internet to overcome this barrier.

This research investigates the effect of these factors on the use of specific technologies such as the Internet, video conferencing and groupware.

Personal factors are the users' attributes, for example, their acceptance of change and attitude towards new technology. Holt (1998, p. 69) has discussed how human factors can hinder the use of available information technology. Attitude to information technology is a likely personal factor that could influence the use of global planning technologies. Many psychologists have theorised attitude as a significant personal attribute that tends to predict behaviour. For instance, Ajzen and Fishbein (1980) concluded in their study that, provided they are appropriately measured, attitudes are sufficient to predict intentions (behaviour). Moghaddam (1998) presents both sides of the research and arguments as to whether attitude predicts behaviour. He tends to conclude that we can use attitude to measure behaviour provided (a) we are relatively specific in our measure; and (b) we measure all the components to provide a better chance of capturing all the facets of the attribute. The components of attitude, which makes operationalisation possible, are cognitive, affective and behavioural. This study measures knowledge of ICT use for global planning (cognitive) and feelings (which includes level of satisfaction) about it (affection), and compares these with actual use (behaviour). The development of questions to measure these components is based on attitude scales developed by Kay (1989), who later used them to predict commitment to use computers (Kay 1990).

Infrastructural factors refer to basic facilities such as electricity and telephone systems, which may be inadequately provided in less developed economies and this inadequacy could therefore hinder the use of global planning technologies (Holt 1998; Barker 1993, pp. 57–59). While availability of supportive telephone systems, including technologies such as ISDN and other broadband transmissions, may present no problem in developed economies, it may not be adequate in developing ones such as South Africa. This inadequacy may present significant problems for the networking aspect of information technology needed for global planning. Big multinationals such as Exxon Mobil in Nigeria provide for these facilities, including electricity and Internet backbone. To what extent can multinationals provide for themselves where the government cannot? The availability of infrastructure and the ability of companies to provide infrastructure by themselves when these are inadequate are examined to investigate their effect on the use of ICT for global planning.

METHODS

The factors expressed in the theoretical model (see above) were operationalised into a questionnaire, copies of which were distributed to a sample of multinational companies in the United Kingdom and South Africa. The sample size was 50 for each country. Only 16 companies responded. Three of the companies apologised that it is against their policy to answer survey questions. One left large areas of the questionnaire uncompleted because according to the respondent, 'I don't believe we use IT as a global planning tool'. This questionnaire was consequently excluded in the analysis to avoid undue bias. It would, however, be very interesting to follow up this respondent with an interview to discover how they carry out international trade in approximately eight countries without using ICT to plan. The analysis performed in this paper is based on the remaining 12 returned questionnaires (12% response rate) and therefore it is best to consider the results as derived from a pilot study. Very interesting observations can be deduced from the returned questionnaires. Correlation analysis and averages (arithmetic means) are used to analyse data collected largely by Likert scale type of questionnaire. Correlation coefficients[9] are widely used in the presentation of the findings.

[9] Correlation coefficients represent relationships of two sets of data at a time. Their values range from −1 (perfect negative correlation) to +1 (perfect positive correlation). The nearer the coefficients are to these two values, the stronger the relationship. The more the coefficients are close to 0, the less the relationship; at 0, there is no relationship.

FINDINGS AND DISCUSSION

The discussion of findings is organised around the major factors that the questionnaire sought to measure. However, use of specific planning technologies is considered first. These technologies are the Internet, intranets, extranets, groupware, enterprising planning tools, video conferencing, data warehousing/mining and others.

Use of ICT in Global Planning

As shown in Figure 5.2, all the respondents use the Internet for strategic planning, and nearly all use video conferencing facilities. Four of the respondents use systems other than those listed on the questionnaire. These, reflected under the 'Others' category in Figure 5.2, are external databases (e.g. Reuters) and others that are not available on the Internet, data collection and analysis applications (e.g. Holos, Hyperion, Market Modeller, Epic) and spreadsheet applications (e.g. Excel and Lotus 123).

Although all respondents use the Internet, for those who own groupware systems, groupware systems are most frequently (daily) used (see Figure 5.3). The Internet and intranets are the next most frequently used systems for global planning. This suggests a great need for collaborative working and external information sourcing in global planning.

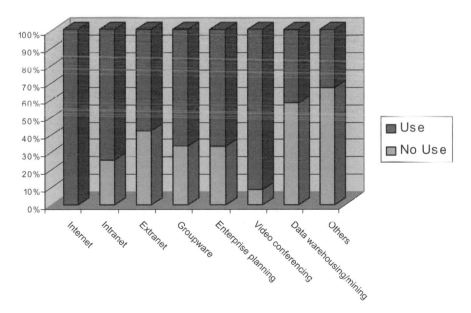

Figure 5.2. Use of information technology

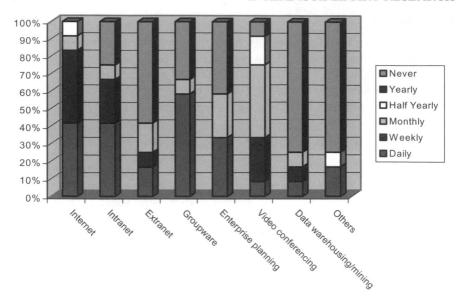

Figure 5.3. Frequency of ICT use

The rest of the findings examine the factors that influence the use of global planning tools.

Organisational Factors

Strategic stance or level of globalisation was operationalised in terms of (a) standardisation of products, services and practices irrespective of country of operation, (b) not exporting 'home' standards to foreign countries and (c) number of countries operated in. These three strands of globalisation as well as involvement in global planning and years in business are discussed below.

Standardisation of Products, Services and Practices

Standardisation of products, services and practices correlates positively (0.31) with the use of ICT for global planning. Since standardisation attenuates variety, it is expected standardisation would increase the use of ICT which itself tends to work well with standard procedures. The increased use does not, however, imply that much original planning or exploration of new opportunities worldwide is taking place, hence the zero correlation between standardisation and involvement in global planning (which was defined as identification of business opportunities irrespective of country). This indicates that ICT for global planning needs to give more support to creativity.

Not Exporting 'Home' Standards to Foreign Countries

A correlation coefficient of -0.18[10] indicated that the more companies use original country standards as *de facto* abroad, the more they use ICT for global planning. Again, this situation suggests less originality and variety to deal with in the planning process. This may not be a problem for some companies in relatively stable industries and markets, but the picture would be different with companies in relatively turbulent industries, with which the present ICT planning tools do not seem adequately able to deal.

Number of Countries Operated in

Surprisingly, there is a negative relationship (-0.038) between number of countries operated in and the use of ICT for global planning. It also appears that the greater the number of countries operated in, the less do the companies adopt a global standard (-0.45) and the more do they use original home country standards (0.19). It therefore appears that the greater the number of countries operated in, the more planning is delegated to individual countries or regions, therefore causing a reduction in overall global planning and use of information technology for that purpose. Also, this result may indicate that very large companies with a presence in a large number of countries are not having adequate help to plan globally.

Years in Business

There is a very high positive relationship (0.7) between the years in business and the use of ICT in global planning. This finding is not surprising in view of the accumulated experience and financial backing, which makes it easier for older organisations to acquire and use the necessary systems.

Involvement in Global Planning

Though not very large, there is a positive relationship (0.008) between involvement in global planning and the use of information technology. It appears the fewer the number of countries operated it, the more the involvement in global planning (-0.05). This may reflect the aim of smaller companies to explore more new opportunities, which was depicted in the definition of involvement in global planning. It is interesting also that companies which tended to be involved in global planning were also not keen on exporting 'home' standards abroad (0.31). The small correlation, though positive, between involvement in global planning and use of ICT probably indicates that inadequate use is made of information technology in global planning.

---

[10] The negative correlation coefficient is between the use of ICT and globalisation as expressed by *not* exporting home standards abroad.

ICT Factors

ICT attributes (see above) were measured. On average the highest four ICT attributes that were found to be important to users are:

(a) provision of timely information;
(b) provision of report and presentation facilities;
(c) support for group working within the same site;
(d) support for group working in more than one site within a country.

These attributes weighted the least:

(a) on-demand link to internal information for indication of company strengths and weaknesses;
(b) access to external data pools – non-company data;
(c) adequate support given for use of systems;
(d) alternative views of information with highly summarised and detailed views.

It is paradoxical that systems that are weak on linking with internal and external data sources are described as providing timely information. This suggests that the timely information is less complete than would be desired, hence the absence of 'provision of complete information' among the top four attributes.

It is interesting to observe that when each of the factors is correlated with the use of information technology, almost all correlate positively. The two exceptions are (a) report and presentation facilities (0.11), and (b) adequate support given for use of systems (0.04). The four top correlated factors, in their order of priority, are:

(a) alternative views of information with highly summarised and detailed views;
(b) on-demand link to internal information for indication of company strengths and weaknesses;
(c) flexibility to solve diverse problems;
(d) access to external data pools – non-company data.

Personal Factors

Cognitive and affective components of attitude were measured and compared to the behavioural component. There is a high positive relationship (0.46) between cognition and affection. This means that the more managers know the capabilities of global planning technologies, the more they feel positive about using them. Satisfaction with the use of global planning technologies was measured as part of affection. Correlating satisfaction with use results in a positive relationship of 0.18, which suggests that we can increase the level of use by increasing level of satisfaction with the systems. The fact that the positive relationship is not very high indicates that managers are not necessarily very happy with the systems they are using. This suggests the need to investigate how to provide more satisfactory systems.

There is surprisingly a negative correlation (−0.34), though not large, between the behavioural component of attitude (use) on the one hand and cognition and affection on the other. This finding is at variance with findings of other studies, such as McGuire and Hillan (1999, pp. 54–55), which propose that cognition (knowledge) should be positively related to behaviour. The smallness of the sample perhaps explains this unexpected result. Otherwise, it may be another case of proof that affective attitude does not always predict behaviour (Moghaddam 1998). Yet another explanation is that managers use the systems more out of necessity than out of affection for them, which suggests that more could be done to improve the experience of using the systems, which improvement consequently should increase their level of use.

Other personal factors that were examined are age, gender, education and experience. Experience exhibits the highest positive relationship (0.41) with use. This result agrees with studies by Walters and Necessary (1996, pp. 623–611) and Igbaria and Chakrabarti (1990, pp. 229–241). Age is the next in the value of positive relationship (0.25). This may be because with age comes experience generally, which is shown in the 0.37 relationship between the two factors. On the other hand, education correlates negatively (−0.33) with use. This result is in contrast with earlier studies by McGuire and Hillan, which found that although the midwives they studied had a positive attitude (feeling) about computers, they considered that lack of the necessary skills as a hindrance to using computers (1999, pp. 54–55), and Igbaria and Chakrabarti, who found computer training to be contributing strongly to a decrease in computer anxiety (1990, pp. 229–241). This contrast might be because the question referred to the level of education rather than its content. It might also mean that the higher the level of education, the less the information technology content. It made no sense to relate gender with the use of information technology because all the respondents were male, tending to confirm that top companies' jobs are still dominated by males. A future study can verify the use by females of global planning tools by the use of quota sampling of respondents.

Infrastructural Factors

As expected (see above), there is a positive correlation (0.2) between the use of ICT for global planning and the provision of infrastructural facilities. The correlation is more pronounced with provision of electricity (0.36) than telephone systems (0.012). The respondents were offered the opportunity to indicate other aspects of infrastructural facilities that may be relevant, but none was indicated. Sometimes, it becomes too expensive for organisations to self-provide the key infrastructures. Hence, some governments of even developing countries such as Singapore have taken the initiative to provide these necessary facilities (Teo & Lim, 1999, pp. 27–36).

Other Findings

The difference between South African and non-South African companies was interesting. On average, use of ICT in global planning by South African companies is 2.5 (arithmetic mean) whereas non-South African multinationals score 3.8, indicating greater use. This outcome suggests that ICT planning tools are used more by UK-based companies than South African companies. The reason for this difference needs further exploration. This result is not conclusive given the small number of respondents upon which the calculations are based. However, a possible explanation is the comparatively lower level of computerisation in developing parts of the world such as Africa (Nkereuwem 1997; Shibanda & Musisi-Edebe, 2000).

MAJOR CONCLUSIONS AND RECOMMENDATIONS

The pilot study aimed at examining the use of global planning tools by multinational companies. The results indicate that the Internet, groupware, enterprise planning and video conferencing tools are very popular. Managers claim that the most important features of ICT for global planning are the provision of timely information, report and presentation facilities, and support for group working. When level of use of global planning tools is compared to view of ICT attributes, other important ICT factors (attributes) emerged, for example, alternative (highly summarised and detailed) views of information.

Another major finding is that managers are not very satisfied with the provision of technology for global planning. This tends to agree with the finding that the information technology they use for global planning does not provide adequate creativity needed in global planning. Besides, there appears to exist the need to improve the experience of using the systems, as borne out with the finding of little or no relationship between affective attitude towards and use of ICT for global planning.

It is the major recommendation of this paper, therefore, that investigation be made on how to use ICT more creatively in global planning. Also, ICT attributes that count highest to managers should be incorporated in any development of computerised global planning tools with a view to improving the use experience, and consequently increase the use, of ICT for global planning.

FURTHER RESEARCH

Further research should examine how to use ICT more creatively in global planning. Moreover, while the major predictor variables of the theoretical model have been derived from secondary research, it is necessary to reconsider and possibly expand the sub-factors. For instance, leadership style could be included within *personal* factors. It has been studied in relation to its effect on the use of strategic tools and models (Drago & Clements 1999, pp. 11–18). Also, *organisational* factors should incorporate the control and regulation of planning process, and the structure of the organisation. Jarvenpaa and Ives (1993, p. 547) discovered a poor fit between organisational structure and global information technologies.

This reworking of the theoretical model and possibly statistical testing of measuring instruments should be performed before further primary data is collected to assess current use of ICT for global planning. Since we are dealing with a moving target, there will be a need to repeat the study from time to time. The repeat studies will also help to further refine the model as well as to compare performance in different parts of the world. In order to improve performance meanwhile, practitioners could note the suggested factors explored in this study and how they influence the use of ICT for global planning as explained in the article.

REFERENCES

Ajzen, I., Fishbein, M. (1980) *Understanding Attitudes and Predicting Social Behaviour.* Prentice Hall, Englewood Cliffs, NJ.

Alkhafaji, A. F. (1991) Management challenges: a worldwide perspective. *Management Decision* June, 29.

Ansoff, H. I. (1979) *Strategic Management.* Macmillan, London.

Avgerou, C. (2005) Doing critical research in information systems: some further thoughts. *Information Systems Journal* **15**, 103–109.

Avison, D., Fitzgerald, G., Powell, P. (2001) Reflections on information systems practice, education and research: 10 years of the *Information Systems Journal. Information Systems* **11**, 3–22.

Backhouse, J., Liebenau, J., Land, F. (1991) On the discipline of information systems. *Information Systems Journal* **1**, 19–27.

Ball, D. A., McCullock, W. H. (1996) *International Business: The Challenges of Global Competition.* Irwin, Chicago, IL.

Barker, R. M. (1993) Information system development in a global environment. *Business Forum* **18**, 57–59.

Buckley, P. J. (1998) A perspective on the emerging world economy: protectionism, regionalisation and competitiveness. In H. Mirza (ed.) *Global Competitive Strategies in the New World Economy* (pp. 12–21). Edward Elgar, Cheltenham.

Business Week (2000) 28 August, i3696, p. 113.

Campbell, D., Stonehouse, G., Houston, B. (1999) *Business Strategy: An Introduction.* Butterworth Heinemann, Oxford.

Carter, H. (1999) Strategic planning reborn. *Work Study* **48**(2), 46–48.

Chae, M. S., Hill, J. S. (1996) The hazards of strategic planning for global markets. *Long Range Planning* **29**, 880–891.

Chakravarthy, B. S., Lorange, P. (1991) Adapting strategic planning to the changing needs of a business. *Journal of Organizational Change Management* **4**(2).

Claver, E., Gonzálex, R., Llopis, J. (2000) An analysis of research in information systems (1981–1997). *Information and Management* **37**, 181–195.

Currie, W. (2000) *The Global Information Society.* John Wiley & Sons, New York.

Davis, G. B. (1999) A research perspective for information systems and example of emerging area of research. *Information Systems Frontiers* **1**, 195–203.

Desai, A. B. (2000) Does strategic planning create value? The stock market's belief. *Management Decision* **38**, 685–693.

Doremus, P. N., Keller, W. W., Pauly, L. W., Reich, S. (1999) The myth of the global corporation. *Harvard Business Review* **77**, 165–171.

Drago, W. A., Clements, C. (1999) Leadership characteristics and strategic planning. *Management Research News* **22**, 11–18.

Feurer, R., Chaharbaghi, K. (1995) Strategy development: past, present and future. *Management Decision* **33**, 11–21.

Fletcher, K., Donaghy, K. (1994) The role of competitor information systems. *Information Management and Computer Security* **2**(3), 4–18.

Fulmer, R. M., Sashkin, M. (1995) Tools for the global learning organization. *American Journal of Management Development* **1**(3), 26–31.

Govindarajan, V., Gupta, A. (2000) Analysis of the emerging global arena. *European Management Journal* **18**, 274–284.

Grant, G. G. (2003) Strategic alignment and enterprise systems implementation: the case of Metalco. *Journal of Information Technology* **18**, 159–175.

Grant, P., Usoro, A. (2003) Herzberg's two-factor theory of motivation following an ERP implementation in a non-commercial organisation. M. G. Hunter & K. K. Dhanda (eds) *ISOneWorld Conference Proceedings, April 23–25, 2003.* The Information Institute, Washington, DC.

Grosse, E. (ed.) (2000) *Thunderbird on Global Business Strategy.* John Wiley & Sons, Toronto.

Hagmann, C., McCahon, C. S. (1993) Strategic information systems and competitiveness: are firms ready for an IST-driven competitive challenge? *Information and Management* **25**, 183–192.

Hamilton, S., Ives, B. (1982) MIS research strategies. *Information and Management* **5**, 339–347.

Harvey, M., Griffith, D., Novicevic, M. (2000) Development of timescopes to effectively manage global inter organizational relational communications. *European Management Journal* **18**, 646–662.

Hax, A. C. (1989) Building the firm of the future. *Sloan Management Review* Spring, 75–82.

Hertzberg, H. (1995) *The Rise and Fall of Strategic Planning.* Prentice Hall, Englewood Cliffs, NJ.

Hill, C. W. L. (1998) *Global Business Today.* McGraw Hill, New York.

Ho, C. (1996) Information technology implementation strategies for manufacturing organizations: a strategic alignment approach. *International Journal of Operations and Production Management* **16**(7), 77–100.

Holt, D. H. (1998) *International Management: Text and Cases.* Dryden Press, London.

Houben, G., Lenie, K., Vanhoof, K. (1999) A knowledge-based SWOT-analysis system as an instrument for strategic planning in small and medium sized enterprises. *Decision Support Systems* **26**(2), 125–135.

Hull, C. W. (1987) Business in a global economy. *Hydrocarbon Processing* December, 61–66.

Humes, S. (1993) *Managing the Multinational: Confronting the Global–Local Dilemma.* Prentice Hall, London.

Ietto-Gillies, G. (1997) Internationalisation trends. In R. John, G. Ietto-Gillies, H. Cox & N. Grimwade *Global Business Strategy* (pp. 73–90). International Thomson Business Press, London.

Igbaria, M., Chakrabarti, A. (1990) Computer anxiety and attitudes towards microcomputer use. *Behaviour and Information Technology* **9**, 229–241.

International Monetary Fund (1997) *World Economic Outlook* (p. 45). IMF, Washington, DC.

Ives, B., Jarvenpaa, S. L., Mason, R. O. (1993) Global business driver: aligning information technology to global business strategy. *IBM Systems Journal* **32**, 143–161.

Jarvenpaa, S. L., Ives, B. (1993) Organising for global competition: the fit of information technology. *Decision Sciences* **24**, 547–581.

Jeannet, J. (1999) Strategies in the spider's web. In *Mastering Global Business* (pp. 28–32). Pitman, London.

Johnson, G., Scholes, K. (1997) *Exploring Corporate Strategy*, 4th edn. Prentice Hall, London.

Kay, J. (1993) The structure of strategy. *Business Strategy Review* **4**(2), 17–37.

Kay, R. H. (1989) A practical and theoretical approach to assessing computer attitudes: the computer attitude measure (CAM). *Journal of Research on Computing in Education* Summer, 456–463.

Kay, R. H. (1990) Predicting student teacher commitment to use of computers. *Journal of Educational Computing Research* **6**, 299–309.

McGrath, K. (2005) Doing critical research in information systems: a case of theory and practice not informing each other. *Information Systems Journal* **15**, 85–101.

McGuire, M., Hillan, E. (1999) Obstacles to using a database in midwifery. *Nursing Times* **95**(3), 54–55.

Moghaddam, F. M. (1998) *Social Psychology: Exploring Universals across Cultures* (pp. 99–129). W. H. Freeman, New York.

Morgan, N. A., Piercy, N. F. (1993) Increasing planning effectiveness. *Management Decision* **31**(4).

Nkereuwem, E. E. (1997) A prescriptive model for planning a national scientific and technical information network for Nigeria. *OCLC Systems and Services* **13**(3), 98–101.

Nolan, R. L., Wetherbe, J. C. (1980) Toward a comprehensive framework for MIS research. *MIS Quarterly*, **4**(2), 1–19.

Ohmae, K. (1989) Managing in a borderless world. *Harvard Business Review* **67**, 152–161.

Özsomer, A., Calantone, R. J., Bonetto, A. D. (1997) What makes firms more innovative? A look at organizational and environmental factors. *Journal of Business and Industrial Marketing* **12**, 400–416.

Penrose, E. T. (1963) *The Theory and the Growth of the Firm.* Blackwell, Oxford.

Quazi, H. A. (2001) Sustainable development: integrating environmental issues into strategic planning. *Industrial Management and Data Systems* **101**(2), 64–70.

Reid, D. M. (1989) Data access and issue analysis in strategic planning. *Marketing Intelligence and Planning* **7**(1).

Rugman, A. M., Hodgetts, R. M. (1995) *International Business and Strategic Management Approach*. McGraw-Hill, New York.

Ryan, T. (1990) Dermatology – global planning in relation to leprosy management. *Leprosy Review* **61**, 209–212.

Sharratt, M., Usoro, A. (2003) Understanding knowledge-sharing in online communities of practice. *Electronic Journal of Knowledge Management*, **1**, paper 18 [online: http://www.ejkm.com/volume-1/volume1-issue-2/issue2-art18-abstract.htm].

Sharratt, M., Usoro, A. (2004) Preliminary result of empirical study of factors affecting knowledge-sharing in online communities. In K. Grant (ed.) *Proceedings of the UKAIS 2004 Conference*. Glasgow Caledonian University, Glasgow. ISBN: 1-903661-56-0.

Shibanda, G. G., Musisi-Edebe, I. (2000) Managing and developing the strategy for Africa's information in global computerization. *Library Management* **21**, 228–235.

Sokol, R. (1992) Simplifying strategic planning. *Management Decision* **30**(7).

Stough, S., Eom, S., Buckenmyer, J. (2000) Virtual teaming: a strategy for moving your organisation into the new millennium. *Industrial Management and Data Systems* **100**, 370–378.

Taggart, J. H., McDermott, M. C. (1993) *International Business*. Prentice Hall, London.

Teo, T. S. H., Lim, V. K. G. (1999) Singapore – an 'intelligent island': moving from vision to reality with information technology. *Science and Public Policy* **26**, 27–36.

Tetteh, E., Burn, J. (2001) Global strategies for SMe-business: applying the SMALL framework. *Logistics Information Management* **14**, 171–180.

Toyne, B., Walters, P. G. P. (1993) *Global Marketing Management: A Strategic Perspective*, 2nd edn. Allyn & Bacon, London.

Truex, D. P., Baskerville, R. (1998) Deep structure or emergence theory: contrasting theoretical foundations for information systems development. *Information Systems Journal* **8**, 99–118.

Uenohara, M. (1992) Innovation on a global scale. *Chemtech* **22**, 402–405.

Usoro, A. (1998) A tool for strategic planning to support managers, 8th Annual BIT (Business Information Technology) Conference, 4/5 November.

Usoro, A. (2001) Can information technology help managers plan globally? *Journal of Global Information Management* **9**, 17–24.

Usoro, A. (2002) The place of ICT in global planning. In F. Tan (ed.) *Advanced Topics in Global Information Management* (pp. 136–149). Idea Group Publishing, London.

Usoro, A. (2005) An exploratory study into dimensioning of culture as a major influence on knowledge-sharing by global virtual teams. In A. Wenn & K. K. Dhanda (eds) *Enabling Executive Information Technology Competencies: ISOneWorld Conference Proceedings, April, 2005*. The Information Institute, Washington, DC.

Usoro, A., Kuofie, H. S. (2006) Conceptualisation of cultural dimensions as a major influence on knowledge sharing. *International Journal of Knowledge Management* **2**(2), 16–25.

Van Horn, R. L. (2973) Empirical studies of management information systems. *Data Base* **5**, 172–180.

Walsham, G. (2005) Learning about being critical. *Information Systems Journal* **15**, 111–117.

Walters, J. E., Necessary, J. R. (1996) An attitudinal comparison towards computers between underclassmen and graduating seniors. *Education* **116**, 623–631.

Wheelen, T. L. (2000) *Strategic Management and Business Policy: Entering 21st Century Global Society*, 7th edn. Prentice Hall, Upper Saddle River, NJ.

Yehia, M., Chedid, R., Ilic, M., Zobian, A., Tabors, R., Lacallemelero, J. (1995) Global planning methodology for uncertain environments – application to the Lebanese power-system. *IEEE Transactions on Power Systems* **10**, 332–338.

6 Hearing Lips and Seeing Voices: Illusion and Serendipity in Auditory-Visual Perception Research

JOHN MACDONALD
Division of Psychology, University of Paisley, UK

INTRODUCTION

The principal issue of this chapter to consider is a particular version of a fundamental issue in psychology. The general issue is what do we know about the objects and events we experience, and how do we arrive at that knowledge? The second aim of the chapter is to consider some of the techniques by which psychologists arrive at an understanding of these psychological processes, and the surprises that can arise in that quest for understanding. All objects we experience have physical and functional properties. A key question that psychologists pose is what does the brain store of the properties of objects? In psychological terms we refer to this as the 'representation' issue. This chapter will restrict this very general question to something rather more specific and describe one particular approach to the study of that question. The general question to be covered here is how do we process speech and what properties of speech does the brain represent?

These issues will be covered by describing some research that I have been involved with, on and off, over the past 25+ years, and the work of other psychologists and speech scientists who have been active in the same area. The key phenomenon is an illusion that I was involved in discovering. In the course of the remainder of the chapter I hope to convince you that this illusion is not just an interesting and unusual finding in psychology, but that it also provides clues and indicators about the fundamental processes involved in speech perception, and more speculatively that it may also provide clues about the origins and development of speech and language.

Also, I want to illustrate one of the methods that psychologists use in order to study perception, the assumptions they make, the strategies adopted etc.

Interdisciplinary Research: Diverse Approaches in Science, Technology, Health and Society.
Edited by J. Atkinson and M. Crowe.
Copyright © 2006 by John Wiley & Sons, Ltd.

This particular approach involves presenting people with stimuli that they would never be exposed to in the natural world and recording their behaviour and/or experience. That is, in order to explore the mechanisms of human perceptual processes, we present the system with unnatural, artificially created stimuli and observe how it copes. The assumption is that the response of the system to these situations will help reveal its operating principles in ways that may not be apparent when using 'natural' stimuli. In brief, the chapter will consider some aspects of the nature of psychological science and enquiry. I will attempt to draw some conclusions and illustrate the potential importance of this research approach for both theory and practice. Finally, I will comment on the serendipitous nature of much scientific enquiry and discovery.

Much of the research described here was carried out in conjunction with Professor Harry McGurk, my PhD supervisor and a research colleague at the University of Surrey. That is where the early research I shall be describing was conducted. The second group of individuals who should be acknowledged are those technicians who responded to requests to do unusual things with audio and videotape materials, particularly those at the Universities of Surrey and Portsmouth. In the early days of this research the audio-visual technology was difficult and time-consuming to operate. Creating the materials took much time and effort. The ability to independently manipulate auditory and visual information was a key component of this research. As will be argued later, greater sophistication in the technology allows even more control over the key variables in the research enterprise. Much scientific progress depends upon developments in technology.

The third group of individuals who deserve thanks are the models used, particularly Sue Ballantyne (the person we used in the original series of studies) and Rachel Seymour (who has acted as model in our recent experiments). Their ability to 'act natural' while producing the required utterances is a difficult task.

UNDERSTANDING PERCEPTION

In general, what we know about the world largely derives from information we receive through our senses – sight, hearing, touch, smell, taste (Coren et al. 1999). Most objects will provide us with some information in many if not all of these senses. For example, if we touch different surfaces, we can discern information about the solidity and texture of objects. Objects can also provide us with information about colour, size, shape, orientation, distance etc. through our visual sense. However, what we inhabit and experience is not a world of disparate sensory information, but a world of objects. One of the basic issues that has occupied psychologists (and philosophers) is how information from our different sensory systems is processed and put together in order to give rise to an integrated perceptual experience of the objects under consideration – the problem of perceptual integration (Bertelson 1998). Rather than consider that very large and general question in this essay, we will restrict discussion to the perception of speech. Speech is obviously a very important aspect of human functioning. Understanding how speech is processed will also give us clues about processing in the other senses.

In the middle to late 1970s the prevailing view was that the development of the senses entailed moving from a position where each sense was processed independently, and that the task for the developing baby was to integrate these independent sources to produce a unified perceptual world (McGurk & MacDonald 1978). What our research entailed was presenting young infants – 3 to 18 months old – with still pictures of objects (people and other objects) and simultaneously playing them sounds (voices or non-speech sounds), measuring how much visual attention they paid to these combinations and trying to decide whether they had come to associate the sound with the visual object presented. The primary assumption was that differential attentional behaviour was indicative of differential processing activity in the mind of the infant. The key methodological strategy was to systematically manipulate the visual and sound relationships of these events, observe what effect this had on the child's behaviour and so uncover what representations the child had of these events. Around 1975 we decided to concentrate on faces and voices and to use dynamic visual stimuli. The development of more easily accessible videotape technology allowed researchers to make their own moving images (mostly black and white). Faces are clearly significant objects in both the adult's and the infant's perceptual and social world (Bruce 1988). Studies had been published showing young infants' abilities to recognise their mother's voice (Mills & Melhuish 1974) and that newborns could imitate some facial gestures (Meltzoff & Moore 1977). Both of these demonstrated that babies of that age were sensitive to the relationship between sight and sound in the first case, and sight and motor (or kinaesthetic) information in the second study.

SPEECH AND AUDIO-VISUAL SPEECH PERCEPTION

What we decided to do was to play infants video clips of a person speaking to them and again monitor their attention. We would construct the clips so that they were either 'congruent' – the face and voice would be saying the same thing – or 'incongruent' – the face and voice would be saying different things. The rationale was to attempt to disrupt the normal relationship between sight and sound for faces and voices and see whether the babies noticed. If the babies responded differently to the 'incongruent' stimuli from the 'congruent' stimuli then that would be evidence that they 'noticed' the difference, in the same way that you and I can 'notice' and feel uncomfortable when we see badly synchronised images on film or television. The question was would the babies pay different amounts of attention to the congruent and incongruent presentations? If they did show differential amounts of attention then this would tell us that they were sensitive to the relationship between the visual and auditory information. Note it does not matter if they pay more attention or less attention to the incongruent stimuli, only that it is different.

In order to do this in a controlled manner we used simple sounds – consonant/vowel combinations – rather than continuous speech, the argument being that these would be easier to control in terms of the onset and offset of the visual and auditory information. These simple sounds are also typical of the speech that adults often use with babies. We video recorded our model saying a selection of sounds called the stop consonants and nasals – 'baba', 'gaga', 'mama' etc. The tapes were taken to the university audio-visual aids unit and they were asked to make up tapes of congruent and incongruent clips as we specified, where a particular speech sound was dubbed either onto a face saying the same sound (congruent) or a different sound (incongruent). When the tapes had been prepared we viewed them and were surprised by what we experienced. It appeared that the audio-visual technicians had not done what had been asked; the speech did not sound right. As we viewed the tapes, we realised that the technicians had done what they had been asked and that we were both hearing the same thing but experiencing an illusion – hearing something that wasn't there. We showed the tapes to others, who also reported the same responses as ourselves. We then decided to run an experiment and asked our participants a simple question for a straightforward task – watch the television screen and report what you hear.

What we found was that the overwhelming majority of people reported something other than the 'sound' presented, and their responses were largely consistent. In this example, when the face is mouthing 'gaga' and the voice is saying 'baba', the report is predominantly 'dada'. You 'hear' something that isn't there. A search of the science literature found nothing like it reported elsewhere. We ran some further experiments with the initial material and further combinations of sounds, and published this very quickly in scientific journals (McGurk & MacDonald 1976; MacDonald & McGurk 1978; MacDonald et al. 1978).

THE 'McGURK' EFFECT

Figure 6.1 shows the basic phenomenon for one set of face/voice combinations. A few years after the first publication in 1976, reports of the illusion started appearing as the 'McGurk effect'. The finding generated a flurry of research, which continues even after 30 years. Much of this research has been centred on trying to understand how the 'visual' information from the facial movements is combined with the acoustic information from the speech sound to produce the percept or experience that people report. That is, what information from the facial movements is picked up, how is it processed and how

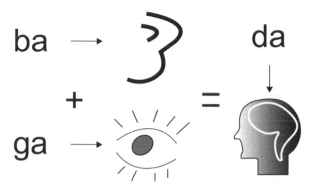

Figure 6.1. An example of the McGurk effect, where audio /ba/ dubbed with video /ga/ results in the heard perception of /da/.

is it used in combination with the auditory information, which would normally be sufficient by itself? In all of our experiments the auditory material is pretested to ensure that participants are able to correctly report the voice when it is presented without the visual information.

Since 1981, Web of Science, the electronic citation index, reports that there have been more than 450 citations of the paper published in *Nature* in 1976. In contrast, another paper that we published in 1978, on the infant work, has had around 50 in the same period. The finding is intriguing and entirely unexpected. It is also something that one cannot imagine being observed without the two important factors: (i) the development of technology that allowed the systematic manipulation and presentation of visual and auditory sources, and (ii) a research approach that sees the use of 'unnatural' events as a technique for uncovering natural processes.

REVIEW OF OTHER STUDIES

Having observed this illusion, the task then becomes one of explaining how and why it occurs. It is not possible here to attempt to review all 450 of these references. What I will do is to review some of the studies and give a flavour of what has been done and found in order to help us understand what is happening in audio-visual speech perception.

Firstly there are some aspects of the visual information that we can change or manipulate that by and large do not affect the occurrence of the illusion. That does not always mean that we can rule these factors out of our explanations. For some we may need to explain why there is no impact.

1. Synthetic faces and voices (Massaro & Cohen 1990; Massaro 1998): using artificial speech and computer generated faces shows the McGurk illusion

when face and voice are mismatched, although typically the level of illusion experienced is not as strong. However, this could be due to the generally greater difficulty in perceiving synthetic speech as compared with the real speech.

2. Mixing gender (Green et al. 1991): dubbing a male voice onto a female face, or vice versa, does not affect the level of illusion. The illusion is still reported in mismatched presentations when gender is also mismatched.

3. Colour or greyscale images (Jordan et al. 2000): whether black and white images are used or colour makes no difference to the level of illusion reported. Most of the original studies used black and white images. More recent studies now tend to use colour images routinely.

4. Being Spanish, Japanese (Massaro et al. 1993) or Finnish (Sams et al. 1998): strong McGurk effects have been reported for some languages, although previous research had found weaker levels of illusion reported (see below).

5. Being young:
   - children (McGurk & MacDonald 1976; Massaro 1984): in the original study (1976) we used children as young as 3–5 years old and a group of 7–8 year olds. The level of illusion reported was lower than that for adults. However, we attributed this to a response bias. The children were more likely to try to report the heard stimulus as a 'real word'.
   - babies (Rosenblum et al. 1997): 5-month-old infants were tested using a habituation paradigm using audio /ba/ and visual /va/ (perceived by adults as /va/), and no difference was found in response from normal audio-visual /va/.

However, there are some factors where manipulation of the stimulus information does substantially affect the level of illusion reported.

1. Being Japanese (Sekiyama & Tohkura 1991) or Chinese (Sekiyama 1997). For these languages very reduced McGurk effects were found. Explaining these rather diverse language results has been problematic. One explanation put forward is that whether or not an illusory response is reported depends upon how common the illusory response is as a syllable in that language. However, it should be noted that in English the syllables /bda/, /namna/, /mna/ are very rare, but are often reported as being 'heard' in some of our mismatched combinations.

2. Face inversion (Green 1994; Jordan & Bevan 1997): presenting the face upside down (or even on different orientations) reduces the illusion (people are much more likely to report the auditory stimulus). This is probably to be expected from typical findings in the face perception literature. People find face recognition and identification much more difficult if the face is presented upside down. Hence in the McGurk conditions with upside down faces, if your face processing mechanisms are disrupted then you are less likely to be influenced by the 'face' aspects of the stimulus.

3. Face familiarity (Walker et al. 1995): if participants know the model used in the study then the McGurk effect is reduced (by about 50%).
4. Mixing the following vowel (Green & Gerderman 1995): for example, if you dub audio /bi/ onto visual /ga/ this produces fewer McGurk illusion type responses than audio /ba/ dubbed onto visual /ga/.

There are a further group of factors that have a graded effect on the level of response reported.

1. Temporal discrepancy (Munhall et al. 1996): varying the onset of the visual and auditory information impacts on the illusion, but the illusion is robust for situations where the audio lags the video by up to 180 milliseconds, i.e. less than 1/5 second. Psychologically, this is a long time in perceptual processing.
2. Point light displays (Rosenblum & Saldana 1996; Jordan et al. 2000): these experiments use small luminous dots placed at strategic points around the face and filmed while saying the speech stimuli. When still, it looks like a set of points; when dynamic one can see it as a 'face'. The percentage of illusory responses is reduced for point light displays (but does not disappear).
3. Brightness reversals (Kanzaki & Campbell 1999): here they reversed the light and dark of the image, like a photographic negative. Again, the illusory effect is reduced but does not disappear.
4. Spatial quantisation (MacDonald et al. 1999, 2000, 2001): finally, there are some recent experiments that I have been carrying out with colleagues (Figure 6.2). As indicated earlier, the traditional view of audio-visual speech perception was one of trying to understand what acoustic information might be extracted from the facial information to be combined with the acoustic – a sort of auditory enhancement assumption. This kind of approach presumes that our perceptual systems engage in some detailed, but yet to be discovered process to uncover information about voicing that

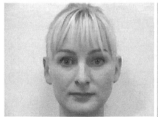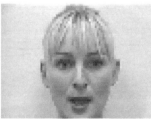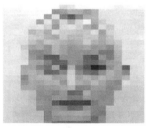

Figure 6.2. Stills of the face stimulus presented under the audio-visual conditions. The first is the original recording, the middle is level 5 (19.4 pixels/face) of the quantisation, and the third is the coarsest quantisation, level 9 (11.2 pixels/face). (*Source:* Department of Psychology, University of Portsmouth).

is then combined with some auditory information to produce the 'heard' percept. However, the research described above suggests that it is increasingly unlikely that the brain engages in processing of minute detail of the face and its movements in order to extract 'acoustic or phonetic' or any other information. Other evidence also suggests that we do not do this. Under normal circumstances we are not able to engage in detailed face processing. For example, although lip movement information helps normally hearing individuals perceive speech in noisy environments, they show limited lip reading ability in visual only conditions (Binnie et al. 1974). Our recent research utilises a technique that allows manipulation of how much detail of the visual information is presented. Hence again we are deliberately creating stimuli that people would not normally experience in order to discover their normal processing capacities. The technique we have used is spatial quantisation (Harmon & Julesz 1973). In effect, the technique allows systematic variation of the amount of detail in the visual information presented.

This spatial quantisation technique is used on television – pixelisation. This is normally used to disguise people's identities or to obscure unsuitable images. This technique is known to affect judgements of facial recognition, the identification of emotion in faces, and visible speech perception (Bachmann 1991; Wallbott 1992; Campbell & Massaro 1997).

The three examples in Figure 6.2 show the end points and the middle of the range of stimuli we used. We used five levels of detail and presented the usual audio-visual matched and mismatched examples. As in previous studies, participants were given the standard instructions of, 'Please watch the television, and tell us what you hear the person saying'. What we found was that the level of illusory responding did vary systematically with the level of quantisation. Figure 6.3 shows one set of results from auditory /ma/ dubbed onto visual /na/ and vice versa. Along the bottom axis is the level of quantisation, from fine to coarse. The vertical axis shows the level of correct auditory responding. At fine levels of visual detail you are affected by the visual information. As the detail

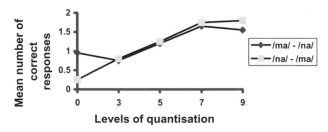

Figure 6.3. Mean number of correct auditory identifications for visual /ma/ with auditory /na/ and for visual /na/ with auditory /ma/ across the levels of spatial quantisation (0 – normal through to 9 – most degraded).

decreases you are less affected. However, for some audio-visual examples people are still affected even at the coarsest level of detail. One way to counteract this pixelisation manipulation is to defocus. Although we observed our participants while they were responding it is possible that some people may have been 'defocusing'.

Hence, from results such as these we conclude that whatever level of information people are using in audio-visual speech perception, it does not require fine levels of detail about the face and lip movements. People are still affected by the visual information even when they can only be picking up fairly gross features of the dynamic properties of the facial movement.

Another question that often arises in this research is what areas or regions of the face are important. The answer that it must be the lips seems self-evident, but we thought that it would be sensible to test that assumption. When people speak, not only is the lip and jaw area in movement but other areas of the face will also be in motion, for example the eyes and forehead.

This suggestion is supported by other findings regarding speech processing and attention. For example, studies of eyetracking (Vatikiotis-Bateson et al. 1998) show that although people do look at the mouth of a speaker in face-to-face interaction, the majority of looking time is spent gazing at the regions around the eyes. At that point, the lips and jaws of the speaker are only in peripheral vision, which again provides much less detailed information than when viewed in foveal (or central) vision.

We have recently carried out some pilot experiments where we have pixelated portions of the face (MacDonald et al. 2001). In one set of conditions, we isolated an area of the face – a box around the lip and jaw region of the face. We then either pixelated the outside of the box and left the lip and jaw region intact, or pixelated the inside of the box and left the outer region of the face intact. We also had a further condition where we varied the size of the box – either all of the lip and jaw region, or only the lip region. What we found was that when you leave the lip and jaw region intact you get strong illusory responses, regardless of what you do to the outside of the face. If you pixelate the lip and jaw region, the level of illusion depends on the degree of quantisation, as in our previous study. Hence, it does seem to be specific information about the speech articulators that is important rather than global dynamic properties of the face. Also, there was very little difference between the lip and the lip and jaw conditions.

IMPLICATIONS FOR SPEECH REPRESENTATION

What, then, are the implications for our understanding of normal speech perception? Does this unnatural and impossible situation tell us anything about how we process everyday speech? Or is it simply an unusual and interesting psychological puzzle with no particular significance?

From the results described above some general principles and conclusions can be drawn. The influence of vision on our perception of speech relies upon fairly crude information from the visual signal (it is fairly robust to some discrepancy – timing, attention, clarity of visual stimulus etc.), but is not immune to gross discrepancy – timing, coarticulation (see vowel mismatch) etc. It does not seem to depend on experience (babies etc.), but is influenced by some experience (the familiarity of the face, the language used).

How, then, does this data about audio-visual speech perception relate to theories of speech perception? Currently there are three major classes of competing theories in speech perception.

PSYCHOACOUSTIC THEORIES

Traditionally, theories of speech perception were formulated to explain auditory speech perception. The dominant approach was to try to explain our perceptual experience by relating it to the physics of the speech sound waves. These are the psychoacoustic theories (Blumstein 1986; Diehl & Kluender 1989). However, these acoustic-based explanations have problems explaining some findings in speech perception. One of these difficulties is that the same speech sound (especially consonants) will have different physical characteristics, not only between different speakers and classes of speakers, but also within speakers. The /d/ of /du/ is different from the /d/ of /di/. To explain the impact of visual information on speech perception, this kind of approach needs to explain how the visual information can be converted into something equivalent to acoustic information to be combined with that from the ears.

MOTOR THEORIES

The major alternative theoretical approach to the psychoacoustic view was the 'motor' theory (Liberman & Mattingly 1985; Mattingly & Studdert-Kennedy 1991). In this account it is proposed that we perceive speech by detecting, from the auditory input, what articulatory gestures produced the stimulus being presented. How that was achieved was rather underspecified in the early version of this theory, which was proposed in the 1960s and predates our 1976 study by a decade or so. However, the 1976 *Nature* paper, which showed an influence of visible speech and facial movements, was eagerly taken up by the 'motor' theorists as strong (and unequivocal support) for their position.

However, although this is intuitively appealing there are some problems with this theory, not the least of which is that there are people who may suffer from speech production disorders but have normal speech perception capabilities (Fourcin 1989). This calls into question the idea of a strong link between perception and production.

DIRECT PERCEPTION

A third theoretical position that has a controversial history in the psychology of perception (Gibson 1979), but has only relatively recently been applied to audio-visual speech perception, is that of 'direct perception' (Fowler 1996). This theory proposes that the function of our sensory systems is to perceive the causes of the sensory input we receive. For example, in the case of speech the cause of the sensory stimulus is the vocal tract activity of the speaker, i.e. what did you do to make that sound? The major challenge for this type of theory was to explain how listeners did this from solely auditory information. This has not been resolved. However, for our purposes this theory has no problem with audio-visual speech perception. Visible speech information simply provides another source of information about the speaker's vocal tract activity.

Clearly there is much further work to be done to distinguish between these theoretical positions. Hence the question of how this illusion comes about (i.e. what processing mechanisms are involved) is still somewhat unresolved.

EVOLUTION OF SPEECH AND LANGUAGE

The idea that speech perception should be thought about more as vocal tract activity, or vocal gesture, rather than a purely acoustic phenomenon is gaining much ground. Professor Michael Corballis, of the University of Auckland, has written about the evolution of speech and language (Corballis 2002). If one views speech as an 'auditory' problem then one might propose that human speech has evolved from animal cries. However, in primates there is a fairly limited repertoire of cries and the vocal apparatus of most primates is limited in range and complexity. In contrast, Corballis has advanced the alternative view that speech and language has evolved not from animal cries and sounds but from gesture. His argument is that this evolution firstly developed through the use of manual gesture. Over the course of evolution this came to include facial expression and facial gesture, primarily for relatively close face-to-face interaction. These gestures would also be accompanied by vocal activity. With associated changes in vocal tract structure and complexity, these visual gestures would be augmented by sounds that would allow a more complex set of sound and speech tokens to be used. Sound, of course, has distinct advantages over visual information – you can use sound at a distance and in the dark, and the listener does not have to be watching you. In this scenario, our current use of visible speech information is viewed as a residue of our evolutionary history. The fact that we often still use facial and manual gesture in our speech and interpersonal communication lends support to this view. The McGurk illusion shows that facial speech information is not simply an adjunct of auditory speech but is an intrinsic component of normal speech perception. This data fits very well with the kind of account that Corballis is putting forward regarding the evolution of speech, and this theory provides an explanation of why we process and are affected by visible speech information and why we experience this illusion.

I hope that I have been able to show and convince you of the value of the research strategy that has underpinned this area of study. At one level it could be argued that this research appears to be the study, in detail, of a rather esoteric piece of behaviour, an illusion that could not occur in real life. Furthermore it has been investigated by a rather unnatural and contrived set of experimental research techniques. From this perspective one might question why so much time and research effort has been expended on the topic. However, my argument is that this is an example of a finding about human sensory processing that could only have been discovered by adopting an approach that attempts to test the limits of human perceptual processing by presenting our sensory systems with stimuli it would not normally encounter and in a controlled and systematic manner. As a result a phenomenon has been observed that, far from being esoteric and inconsequential, has relevance to a fundamental aspect of what makes us human – our advanced and well-developed system of communication, of which speech is one of the more important components. However, a note of caution needs to be introduced. As was argued above, this approach to investigation has been dependent upon technology that allows the manipulation and control of the sensory components of the stimuli used. The methodological danger is that the research enterprise then gets taken over by the methodological and experimental techniques. That is, the stimulus situations and studies are designed and constructed because they can be done, rather than being driven by theoretical considerations. Ultimately this could lead to a rather 'suck it and see' approach to research. Herein lies the tension between research motivated by strong theoretical considerations, articulating clear predictions, and research as exploration where it may be unclear what is to be found, or why it is being done.

Finally, I must comment on the role of serendipity in the research process. The initial phases of these studies were all conducted in line with the hypothetico-deductive approach to scientific endeavour. The rationale and arguments for the experiments were a result of systematic examination of previous theory and research, and appropriate predictions made about the possible outcomes, in this case about infant attentional behaviour. However, the important outcomes of the studies, the 'illusory' responses, were not predicted and were entirely unexpected. Even science sometimes relies on luck and chance.

REFERENCES

Bachmann, T. (1991) Identification of spatially quantised tachistoscopic images of faces: how many pixels does it take to carry identity? *European Journal of Cognitive Psychology* **3**, 87–103.

Bertelson, P. (1998) Starting from the ventriloquist: the perception of multimodal events. In M. Sabourin, F. I. M. Craik & M. Robert (eds) *Advances in Psychological Science, II: Biological and Cognitive Aspects* (pp. 419–439). Psychology Press, Hove.

Binnie, C. A., Montogomery, A. A., Jackson, P. L. (1974) Auditory and visual contributions to the perception of consonants. *Journal of Speech and Hearing Research* **17**, 619–630.

Blumstein, S. E. (1986) On acoustic invariance in speech. In J. S. Perkell & D. H. Klatt (eds) *Invariance and Variability in Speech Processes* (pp. 178–197). Lawrence Erlbaum Associates, Hillsdale, NJ.

Bruce, V. (1988) *Recognising Faces.* Lawrence Erlbaum Associates, Hove.

Campbell, C. S., Massaro, D. W. (1997) Perception of visible speech: influence of spatial quantization. *Perception* **26**, 627–644.

Corballis, M. C. (2002) *From Hand to Mouth: The Origins of Language.* Princeton University Press, Princeton, NJ.

Coren, S., Ward, L. M., Enns, J. T. (1999) *Sensation and Perception.* Harcourt Brace, New York.

Diehl, R. L., Kluender, K. R. (1989) On the objects of speech perception. *Ecological Psychology* **1**, 121–144.

Fourcin, A. J. (1989) Links between voice pattern perception and production. In B. A. Elsendoorn & H. Bouma (eds) *Working Models of Human Perception* (pp. 67–91). Academic Press, London.

Fowler, C. A. (1996) Listeners do hear sounds, not tongues. *Journal of the Acoustical Society of America* **99**, 1730–1741.

Gibson, J. J. (1979) *The Ecological Approach to Visual Perception.* Houghton Mifflin, Boston, MA.

Green, K. P. (1994) The influence of an inverted face on the McGurk effect. *Journal of the Acoustical Society of America* **95**, 3014.

Green, K. P., Gerderman, A. (1995) Cross-modal discrepancies in coarticulation and the integration of speech information: the McGurk effect with mismatched vowels. *Journal of Experimental Psychology: Human Perception and Performance* **21**, 1409–1426.

Green, K. P., Kuhl, P. K., Meltzoff, A. N., Stevens, E. B. (1991) Integrating speech information across talkers, gender, and sensory modality: female faces and male voices in the McGurk effect. *Perception and Psychophysics* **50**, 524–536.

Harmon, L. D., Julesz, B. (1973) Masking in visual recognition: effects of two-dimensional filtered noise. *Science* **180**, 1194–1197.

Jordan, T. R., Bevan, K. (1997) Seeing and hearing rotated faces: influence of facial orientation on visual and audio-visual speech recognition. *Journal of Experimental Psychology: Human Perception and Performance* **23**, 388–403.

Jordan, T. R., McCotter, M., Thomas, S. (2000) Visual and audiovisual speech perception with colour and gray-scale facial images. *Perception and Psychophysics* **62**, 1394–1404.

Kanzaki, R., Campbell, R. (1999) Effects of facial brightness reversal on visual and audiovisual speech recognition. Paper presented at the Audio Visual Speech Processing Conference, University of California, Santa Cruz.

Liberman, A. M., Mattingly, I. G. (1985) The motor theory of speech perception. *Cognition* **21**, 1–33.

MacDonald, J., McGurk, H. (1978) Visual influences on speech perception processes. *Perception and Psychophysics* **24**, 253–257.

MacDonald, J., Dwyer, D., Ferris, J., McGurk, H. (1978) A simple procedure for accurately manipulating face-voice synchrony when dubbing speech onto videotape. *Behaviour Research Methods and Instrumentation* **10**, 845–847.

MacDonald, J., Andersen, S., Bachmann, T. (1999) Hearing by eye: visual spatial degradation and the McGurk effect. In G. Olaszy, G. Nemeth & K. Erdohegyi (eds) *Proceedings of Eurospeech '99* (vol. 3, pp. 1283–1286). European Speech Communication Association, Bonn.

MacDonald, J., Andersen, S., Bachmann, T. (2000) Hearing by eye: how much spatial degradation can be tolerated? *Perception* **29**, 1155–1168.

MacDonald, J., Andersen, S., Bachmann, T. (2001) Read my lips, but not too closely: what face information is used in the perception of speech? XII ESCOP and XVIII BPS Cognitive Section Conference, Edinburgh, September.

Massaro, D. W. (1998) *Perceiving Talking Faces. From Speech Perception to a Behavioral Principle.* Bradford/MIT Press, Cambridge, MA.

Massaro, D. W., Cohen, M. M. (1990) Perception of synthesized audible and visible speech. *Psychological Science* **1**, 55–63.

Massaro, D. W., Tsuzaki, M., Cohen, M. M., Gesi, A., Heredia, R. (1993) Bimodal speech perception: an examination across languages. *Journal of Phonetics* **21**, 445–478.

Massaro, M. M. (1984) Children's perception of visual and auditory speech. *Child Development* **55**, 1777–1788.

Mattingly, I. G., Studdert-Kennedy, M. (eds) (1991) *Modularity and the Motor Theory of Speech Perception.* Lawrence Erlbaum Associates, Hillsdale, NJ.

McGurk, H., MacDonald, J. (1976) Hearing lips and seeing voices. *Nature* **264**, 746–748.

McGurk, H., MacDonald, J. (1978) Auditory-visual co-ordination in the first year of life. *International Journal of Behavioral Development* **1**, 229–239.

Meltzoff, A. N., Moore, M. K. (1977) Imitation of facial and manual gestures by human neonates. *Science* **198**, 75–78.

Mills, M., Melhuish, E. (1974) Recognition of mother's voice in early infancy. *Nature* **252**, 123–124.

Munhall, K. G., Gribble, P., Sacco, L., Ward, M. (1996) Temporal constraints on the McGurk effect. *Perception and Psychophysics* **58**, 351–362.

Rosenblum, L. D., Saldana, H. M. (1996) An audio-visual test of kinematic primitives for visual speech perception. *Journal of Experimental Psychology: Human Perception and Performance* **22**, 318–331.

Rosenblum, L. D., Schmuckler, M. A., Johnson, J. A. (1997) The McGurk effect in infants. *Perception and Psychophysics* **59**, 347–357.

Sams, M., Manninen, P., Surakka, V., Helin, P., Katto, R. (1998) McGurk effect in Finnish syllables, isolated words, and words in sentences: effects of word meaning and sentence context. *Speech Communication* **26**, 75–87.

Sekiyama, K. (1997) Cultural and linguistic factors in audiovisual speech processing: the McGurk effect in Chinese subjects. *Perception and Psychophysics* **59**, 73–80.

Sekiyama, K., Tohkura, Y. (1991) McGurk effect in non-English listeners: few visual effects for Japanese subjects hearing Japanese syllables of high auditory intelligibility. *Journal of the Acoustical Society of America* **90**, 1797–1805.

Vatikiotis-Bateson, E., Eigsti, I. M., Yano, S., Munhall, K. G. (1998) Eye movement of perceivers during audiovisual speech perception. *Perception and Psychophysics* **60**, 926–940.

Walker, S., Bruce, V., O'Malley, C. (1995) Facial identity and facial speech processing: familiar faces and voices in the McGurk effect. *Perception and Psychophysics* **57**, 1124–1133.

Wallbott, H. G. (1992) Effects of distortion of spatial and temporal resolution of video stimuli on emotion attributions. *Journal of Nonverbal Behavior* **16**, 5–20.

7 Research in Modern History

MARTIN MYANT

Centre for Contemporary European Studies, University of Paisley, UK

INTRODUCTION

This contribution covers a piece of historical research on political, social and economic development in Czechoslovakia in the period 1945 to 1948. It was started in 1972, leading to a PhD in 1978 and to the publication of a book (Myant 1981). This was reviewed in the appropriate academic journals, with comments ranging from 'the fullest and best-documented study to have appeared in English' (Pravda 1982) to 'seriously flawed' (Ulč 1982). It has been used and commented on in other publications and finds a place as supplementary reading in a number of university courses around the world. Time has passed since then, political constraints have altered, more sources have become available and a number of further important works have been published on related themes. The aim here is to look back on the research and the methods that were used, seeking common features with other kinds of research.

The piece starts with a fairly bland outline of the topic followed by a discussion of how historical research relates to the development of knowledge in general, continuing through a discussion of debates about the nature of history to a consideration of the mechanics of the research. Arguments are then illustrated with a description of how some points, both of detail and of general interpretation, were handled, leading to a concluding section that assesses, in the light of subsequent publications, whether all the effort involved really did lead to an 'original contribution to knowledge'.

THE TOPIC

In very broad outline, the period saw Czechoslovakia emerge from World War II with a coalition government. There were four Czech parties – the National Socialists, the People's Party, the Social Democrats and the Communists – and two Slovak parties, the Democratic Party and the Communists. These six

Interdisciplinary Research: Diverse Approaches in Science, Technology, Health and Society.
Edited by J. Atkinson and M. Crowe.
Copyright © 2006 by John Wiley & Sons, Ltd.

parties formed the 'National Front' and no parties outside that structure were allowed. They were all nominally committed to a programme of revolutionary social and economic changes that communists had previously considered incompatible with a framework of political pluralism. This included international reorientation towards close alliance with the Soviet Union – the West was widely seen as having failed the country with the Munich agreement of 1938 – nationalisation of almost all of industry and the expulsion of the substantial German minority. Elections in 1946 confirmed the Communists as the largest party, with 40% of the Czech and 30% of the Slovak votes, making 38% overall, and the same coalition continued under the Communist Prime Minister Klement Gottwald. President Edvard Beneš was closer to the National Socialists, but tried to stand above party politics.

From mid-1947 the coalition was gripped by increasingly deep divisions over a wide range of internal policy issues, with the Communists either standing alone or backed only by the Social Democrats. Division led to the February crisis of 1948 when the ministers of the remaining three parties offered their resignations in protest at the failure by the Communist Minister of the Interior to implement a government decision reversing personnel changes in the police force. The Communists portrayed this as an attempt to remove them from government and thence to reverse the direction of post-1945 policies. They mobilised mass support and exploited the positions of power they held to establish an effective monopoly of power. This was achieved by nominally constitutional means. The key event was President Beneš's acceptance of a new government under firm Communist domination.

The period has been covered from a number of different points of view. The most numerous sources in the West have been memoirs and accounts by participants who emigrated in 1948. Their aim was often to convince others of a political point of view rather than an open-minded search after 'truth'. Some make efforts to be objective and reflective, but this often relates to the limited issue of exactly what happened in February when resignations, intended to press claims that the Communists wanted to impose a totalitarian regime, opened the easiest possible route to that outcome. This blunder is sometimes explained away with condemnations of the Communists for cunningly concealing their true aims behind claims of allegiance to democracy. Another common theme is to blame Beneš for accepting the ministers' resignations. Beneš's own judgement, as has emerged from a combination of memoir and archival sources, was that he had little choice in view of the weight of public opinion and of a perceived Communist willingness to resolve the issue by force if they felt the need.

Within Czechoslovakia work on the period fell into several periods. In the early 1950s it was dominated by the assumption that February had been a great and definitive victory and by attempts to fit the events into preconceived schemas derived from Marxist writing on the Russian revolution. This was a political necessity – to prove the country's conformity to the then current Soviet intellectual climate – and it led to works contributing nothing of value.

By the 1960s a more reflective approach emerged, with questioning of whether there were not fruitful alternatives that could have led to a more 'democratic' model of socialism. Here at last was research seeking to answer important questions rather than just fitting facts into a preconceived framework.

It became increasingly clear that the Communists were at least partly to 'blame' for ending a possible experiment in democratic socialism, and the first serious questions were asked about whether February 1948 really was a great victory that should be celebrated. The research behind this benefited from access to unpublished sources in state and party archives, but the development of thinking was still incomplete. Ideas imposed by those in power had been questioned, but a completely new framework, which would at least implicitly have challenged the justification for the one-party state, was yet to emerge.

The invasion of Czechoslovakia by Soviet and other Warsaw Pact troops in August 1968 ended the reform movement of the time and, within a few months, also ended official tolerance for the line of historical research referred to above. Published works in the 1970s could not completely ignore what had gone before, and reflected some wider access to archival material, but there was no more writing that could hint at possible alternatives to the Soviet 'model'.

Research on this area could therefore start from a rich body of secondary literature, bringing both factual information and open questions. It could be classified as 'historical' research, simply because it relates to the past. It could also be seen as work covering a number of social science disciplines that happens to relate to a period before the time of writing. However, a number of important characteristics, amplified in the following section, link it more clearly to historical, rather than other kinds of, research.

HISTORY AND KNOWLEDGE IN GENERAL

At one time it was widely accepted that knowledge developed from observation, followed by induction and the formulation of theories. This has been successfully challenged from a number of angles. Popper saw research starting from theories that then lead to testable propositions, after which choice can be made between competing theories (Popper 1994, p. 141). Kolb's (1984) influential notion of experiential learning sees knowledge developing not through the accumulation, assimilation or verification of facts, but through a cyclical process made up of concrete experience, reflective observation, abstract conceptualisation and active experimentation, after which the same cycle can be repeated with a higher level of understanding. We formulate interpretations, test them out, maybe become tied to them, but maintain 'partial skepticism' (Kolb 1984, p. 108): every statement must therefore remain 'tentative forever' (Popper 1959, p. 280). Without that degree of scepticism, we would be unable to develop knowledge further. If it were total, we would not have a starting point for further enquiry.

This kind of cyclical, or spiral, process can be applied across many areas of academic enquiry. A common form for a PhD appears close to a structure explicitly recommended by Popper (1994, p. 106). Existing 'knowledge' is reviewed to reveal gaps. Questions are then posed leading to hypotheses. These are then tested, using data that is either generated by the researcher or found from some other source. The results may lead to conclusions changing the body of knowledge, after which the same process can be repeated. However, behind this general form lie substantial differences in the relative weights attached to different parts of the cycle and the relationships between them.

A starting point for recognising the distinctiveness of historical research is the volume and nature of data. The bibliography from my PhD includes 451 books and 85 newspapers and periodicals, all referred to at some point in the work. A rough estimate suggests well over 200 million words, culminating in a PhD of 150000 words and then a book of under 95000 words. Thus the process involved producing a piece of written work several orders of magnitude smaller than the starting material.

Despite this volume of data, it is necessarily incomplete. A great deal more existed in written form, but access to archives in 1975, when the work inside Czechoslovakia was conducted, was a practical impossibility. At least some of this had been studied by Czechoslovak historians and was available in secondary sources, but it had been filtered through the selection process referred to above. There anyway were still major gaps, most notably in the absence of any information on the contents of Soviet archives. Moreover, some issues may, quite deliberately, have been resolved by word of mouth, leaving no written records.

In some forms of research data can be generated by the researcher. When dealing with past events, we are largely stuck with what the past has left us. There is some scope for bending this for the recent past by speaking to participants, but any formal interviews seemed a practical impossibility in the political conditions of 1975. There anyway are serious dangers in relying too heavily on individual memories, which can be very imprecise. That said, the research was undoubtedly helped by numerous less formal conversations, possibly with hundreds of individuals. They gave general impressions and provided pointers that could be investigated in published sources. Thus they helped pose the questions, but could not be relied on to provide the answers.

These points mean that historical research is heavily dependent on searching out, selecting and manipulating data to produce a finished work, as described in some detail below. This contrasts with the experimental sciences, where data are generated by the researcher using a transparent and repeatable method which, it is assumed, should always produce identical results. Some kinds of research use data from questionnaires and/or surveys, again generated by the researchers and using a transparent methodology. Where appropriate sampling is involved, repetition is expected to lead to similar, but not identical, results. There may also be a substantial data-manipulation process, perhaps involving sophisticated statistical techniques, but the methodology should again be easy to follow.

The methods required for historical research are themselves far less transparent, a point taken up below. There is anyway less scope for such precision. The plausibility of a 'fact' depends less on its independent verifiability – that can be only provisional – than on its consistency with other 'provisionally established' facts. There is thus a much more continuous confrontation of individual points of data with generalisations, interpretations and an overall framework. Relating this back to the cyclical process, there is continuous interaction between the points round the cycle. In other fields of research, data generation and manipulation may become substantially autonomous processes.

This may seem alien to practitioners of experimental sciences, where the practical content of work may appear geared towards precise verification or refutation of identifiable and manageable propositions. However, it is well represented in serious studies of the broad development of scientific knowledge (Lambert & Brittan 1997). It has obvious common ground with the development of interpretations of the world's past in geology and biology, in which data had to be sought out and interpreted. Grand theories were formulated – for example, on the past ice ages – and gained acceptance (Calspace 2002), not so much from key facts that could be proven in any completely conclusive way as from the consistency with which a wide range of phenomena could gain credible explanation and from consistency with other theories and phenomena in apparently diverse scientific disciplines. It can be added that research was not a matter of unstructured observation alone; it was guided and in a sense constrained by broad theories under debate at the time. This has much in common with the method in historical research.

The analogy can be clarified further with reference to Kuhn's (1962, 2000) account of 'scientific revolutions'. He has been widely criticised for exaggerating the extent to which scientific advance depends on battles between adherents to different 'paradigms' who could not communicate, appearing to speak different languages and completely misunderstanding each others' arguments. However, Kuhn appears close to the mark in history, where different interpretations can, as in the case of Czechoslovakia in the 1945–8 period, survive and compete from different political environments. Paradigm shift, or dialogue across paradigms, therefore depends on overcoming political constraints.

It can be added that the nature of much historical research, with the intensity of interaction between the different stages in the cycle, gives much of it the look of a 'scientific revolution', overthrowing a previous general interpretation, rather than as the 'normal science', filling in gaps within an established framework, that Kuhn sees as typical for research. It all makes it much harder to be certain of conclusions and of the objectivity of the historian who has reached them.

CAN HISTORY BE OBJECTIVE?

My intention was to achieve something approaching 'objectivity'. E. H. Carr's 14-volume history of the creation and early years of the Soviet Union directly influenced my conception of how to undertake historical research, and his *What is History?* (Carr 1961), the only work on historical methodology that I knew at the time, served as an ever-present warning of the difficulty of achieving objectivity. It has occupied a central place in debates about the nature of historical research.

A convenient starting point is Carr's discussion of the 'historical fact'. He used an incident in 1850 to demonstrate a distinction between what happened and what happened that might be of interest to a historian. A 'fact' only becomes a 'historical fact' when it is incorporated into a historian's account as part of an argument which is then 'accepted by other historians as valid and significant' (p. 7). It can be added that that argument, built up from generalisations derived from an interpretation of evidence, in turn reflects the questions the historian has posed. In other words, it may reflect biases of time and place and even individual prejudices.

One interpretation of this, following 'postmodern' thinking, is to deny the possibility of objectivity (e.g. Munslow 1997). Thus, Hayden White (1973) has suggested that writing 'history' and writing 'fiction' have much in common. The former appears to require 'finding' rather than 'inventing' facts, but the process of selection and interpretation means that the same set of events can be incorporated into 'a number of equally comprehensive and plausible, yet apparently mutually exclusive, conceptions' (White 1973, p. 41). There are, then, 'no extra-ideological grounds' for deciding between them (p. 26).

Much of historical writing fits closely with White's arguments. Many works have been produced not to report research into unanswered questions, but explicitly to provide persuasive arguments for preconceived positions. They may pay tribute to heroes of the past, or perhaps inform a new generation of a nation's, or political movement's, proud past. However, although there is no clear dividing line, a general distinction can be made between such writing and works that take account of diverse existing views and try to use evidence to choose between competing interpretations. Carr's own work, using enormous numbers of published sources, is consistent with the view that knowledge is always provisional, but that it is worth trying to get closer to 'truth' through careful work. This may be harder than in some other fields of knowledge, but that does not make the exercise pointless.

There is an alternative, 'traditionalist' approach, analogous to the once-popular account of scientific advances via observation and induction. The need is allegedly for an 'exhaustive and exhausting' review of all conceivably relevant documentary evidence (Elton 1967, p. 66), free from constraints allegedly imposed 'from outside', by 'ideological theory' or 'predetermined explanatory frameworks' (Elton 1991, p. 27). This apparently requires skills and methods so specific as to give history the status of 'an autonomous discipline with its own specialised methods' (Marwick 2001, p. 17).

In terms of the cyclical process outlined above, this would seem to obscure the mutual interactions between data gathering and selection and different levels of interpretation. The analogy with researching the world's past is also obscured: theories of past ice ages, of the movements of continents or of the evolution of species were developed from meticulous searches for data, but the searches were structured by theories that had led to the formulation of questions.

Some research might start purely from raw data, but that could not be the case for mine. The method there had to respect the points covered above concerning the volume, diversity and incompleteness of data, the existence of sharply conflicting interpretative frameworks, and the desire to seek general conclusions rather than to check some identifiable points of fact.

The point, then, was to avoid any pretence that it is possible to eliminate preconceptions or to rely on an unstructured assault on primary sources. It was rather to start with as many biases, or rather hypotheses, as possible, all to be pursued when looking through the material. The advice for 'meticulous examination' (Marwick 2001, p. 272) makes sense only when the examination is structured by an idea of what should be sought.

The question of the place of 'theory', taken here to mean the need to start from general interpretations, seems often to be confused with the distinct issue of the possibility of an overarching framework for history in general. Marwick and Elton seem to interpret all considerations of theory around accusations directed against 'Marxists' for allegedly starting from preconceived schemas into which they fit appropriate facts, leaving out, or perhaps not even noticing, any evidence that might point in another direction. This is a valid criticism of some Marxist writing, such as that referred to above produced in Czechoslovakia in the 1950s. Marx, of course, can be quoted arguing against creating a grand historical–philosophical theory and finding 'facts' that fit into it (Carr 1961, p. 59).

Carr addresses the problem in a slightly different way. He relates 'objectivity' to a historian's 'capacity to project his vision into the future' to enable a 'more lasting insight into the past' (Carr 1961, p. 117). Thus, accepting that we ask questions about the past deriving from the present, good history should start with questions that will be relevant in the future. Thus his sympathy for the Soviet planned economy, and his belief that it somehow represented 'progress', led him to concentrate on the 'winners' (Carr 1961, pp. 120–121) who had contributed most to the evolution of the system. He devoted little space to speculating on where alternatives might have led, a point on which he has been strongly criticised (e.g. Evans 1997). By the 1990s the winners seemed to have changed and questions that looked to Carr like idle speculation appeared more interesting. That looks like a warning for keeping a more open mind on varied possibilities for the future when setting the questions for 'interrogating' the past.

It can be added that bias also takes a more personal form. Thus Carr's apparent predilection for 'siding' with the winners, leading to dismissals, for example, as 'that awful old Stalinist and Cambridge snob' (Marwick 2001, p. 3), has also been linked to his experience working in the Foreign Office from 1916 to 1936. Perhaps this taught him not to question decisions after they had been taken or to worry over ideas that did not contribute to policy decisions.

This can be taken further. One's background and experience of life must affect one's ability to understand the actors on the historical stage. Thus, at the apparently trivial level, a judgement has to be made on whether someone is joking, being ironic, embarrassed, exaggerating an issue for dramatic effect and much more beside. This all serves to emphasise the wisdom in Carr's advice to 'study the historian', including the 'historical and social environment', before 'you study the history' (Carr 1961, p. 38). The point is often quoted with approval, although it is still not customary for historians to begin by what could be seen as implicitly confessing sources of potential bias. It would certainly seem odd in other branches of knowledge, where the processes of selecting and manipulating data should be so transparent as to mean that different individuals will always produce the same results.

THE MECHANICS OF RESEARCH

My initial motives and interests included sympathy for the notion that socialism and pluralist democracy could, or rather should, coexist. The work therefore relates to themes that have significance beyond just Czechoslovak history and certainly beyond the period itself. There are obvious points of contact with the subsequent attempt to reform the Communist system 'from within' in the late 1960s and with the country's older democratic traditions. I would probably have been happier researching the social, economic and political developments in the post-1948 period, especially around 1968, leading towards conclusions on the nature and future of the system of the time. Detailed work on that was a practical impossibility. I had to settle for the most recent period that could be researched from reasonably reliable and accessible published sources.

The practical starting point was the formulation of possible frameworks and general hypotheses, using the existing literature. These relate to a wide range of levels of generality, from what lay behind major breaks in development to accounts of apparently relatively minor points of detail. Nevertheless, they all interrelate in one way or another to building the overall picture.

This could appear as a typical 'literature review' stage, familiar in much of social science research. It took a long time – probably well over a year, albeit with some overlap with the next stage – but has practically no presence in the finished work, producing only about 200 words in the book. This is common in works on historical themes, perhaps reflecting times when 'history' differed even less from 'fiction'. It still makes sense as generalisations can often be put in few words and because information from secondary sources is best embodied in the writing of the whole work. So a full review of what others had written – and maybe also why they wrote it – would mean repeating the same ground from numerous angles that were then to be rejected. Instead, the final work comes out as a narrative, in the sense of a roughly chronological account that tells a 'story', with references to secondary sources and other views as appropriate along the way.

The result from this stage was an awareness of alternative interpretations – some of the key questions were easy to identify – but also of some serious gaps. Not enough seemed to have been written on how the economic system functioned or on how it was evolving, or on how different groups in society were affected by, or responded to, the changes that took place after 1945. In short, political changes had been viewed in isolation from other elements of social transformation: these were also areas relevant to a possible alternative 'model' of socialism. There were only a few starting points, such as one work by Karel Kaplan referred to below.

The second stage was the search through material published in the period. All the legal parties produced daily papers, providing a helpful means for checking objectivity, and also a range of further publications. There were some nominally independent papers, specialist journals and publications from factories and local communities. I adopted a blunderbuss approach, using the catalogue in the National Library to find any periodical from the period that might be helpful. The task then was to look for anything that could confirm, refute or develop further, interpretations that had already been identified, or that could fill in gaps that had been identified.

Much of this was done in Prague during nine months in 1975. The time and the place forced an undesirable partial separation of this from the preceding and subsequent stages and imposed certain further constraints. The work amounted to looking through the available material, following key themes from all available viewpoints. I made copious notes on cards – about 3500 in total with around 1 million words of writing – often appending comments as to significance, conflicts with other views and the like. This was an opportunity for continually testing hypotheses, confronting and adapting interpretations. In quantitative terms, it was the most important part of the data-selection process, but there could be no written account of how the selection was undertaken. Although at times tedious, it could be quite a relaxing and enjoyable process. More stressful parts were to come later.

This confrontation with primary sources led almost immediately to questioning of hypotheses. Reality consistently appeared to be more complex than previous works had suggested. Thus, for example, the daily press in May 1945 left little doubt that parties were well aware of how far they differed and of how difficult cooperation could be. Suggestions that the National Socialists and others were somehow tricked into trusting the Communists' democratic credentials sat uneasily alongside their own frequent complaints about 'totalitarianism' or 'Communist terror'. In this sense, as Marwick suggests, the sources could appear to be throwing up new questions, but they were questions that followed from a confrontation of hypotheses with sources.

The search for material on changes in the economic system was also influenced by ideas derived from outside the primary sources. Thus, for example, I pursued anything I could find on factory councils, organs that emerged in 1945 and played a role in the events of February 1948. I was interested in their relationship to political power, but also in their possible role as part of a more participatory model of social organisation and/or of a more decentralised economic system, still based on state ownership. Apparently similar bodies emerged in 1968 and the idea of such autonomous employee organisation had attracted a lot of interest in left-wing circles at that time. It was natural to follow it up as vigorously as possible and that meant a determined trawl through very diverse sources.

In other areas too, the search through sources was structured by almost any available theories and interpretations, inevitably coming from 'outside' the period. Marxist theory, in the broadest sense of a view that history is ultimately dependent on the development of a 'mode of production', had no practical relevance to my research. At a lower level of abstraction, ideas of social classes pursuing their interests seemed well worth investigating. From a different perspective, Hayek's (1944) arguments on the incompatibility of state ownership and political democracy seemed worth following up. They even surfaced in some political propaganda, but it became fairly clear that the processes he predicted had not emerged.

Although 'pure' historians have cautioned against 'too careful an ear cocked for the pronouncements of non-historians' (Elton 1967, p. 25), meaning social scientists, my approach meant that the study of past events is structured by, and serves as a test of, a wide range of theories from apparently diverse disciplines. This appears consistent with the development of knowledge on the world's past, as referred to above.

The third stage involved a more active interaction between data and generalisations, leading to more decisive revision of hypotheses, formulation of new ones and reflection on their interrelationships. This, as already indicated, was under way from the start, but became more central after the principal 'data-collection' stage had reached its forced end. I started by rearranging my cards by theme and then formulated drafts for parts of the final work. I started this process while in Prague and spent maybe another six months on it before firmly embarking on the next stage. This got more difficult, involving worry over issues such as the consistency of arguments, the interpretation of data and the accuracy and completeness of records.

The 'writing-up' stage ultimately determined which bits of evidence would be used and how they would be organised. It took six months for a first draft. That went to my supervisor, who returned substantial comments some weeks later, and the final version, very substantially altered, took about another six months to complete and type.

It is noteworthy that, unlike some other kinds of research, there is no necessary boundary between a research stage and a writing-up stage. This latter is the time when the final decisions have to be made. It is therefore the most stressful, requiring the most concentrated effort. Indeed, a further 'writing-up' stage was required, taking several more months, to convert the PhD into an appropriate form for publication as a book. That required abbreviation and, above all, elimination of numerous sections that discussed the significance of points and that recorded reservations and open questions. The finished product is strongly influenced by the interest in the possibility of alternatives to what did happen, but it had to take the form, as Carr advises (1961, p. 92), 'of explaining what did happen and why', rather than speculating on what might have been. Everything had to find a place in a narrative, creating a work that someone might have the patience to read.

THE OVERALL STRUCTURE

The most central decision in the writing-up phase was the overall structure of the final narrative. This focused on the course and outcome of the central political struggle. That reflected the availability of primary sources and the volume of pre-existing secondary literature that had left a string of claims and unanswered questions. It also reflected the objective fact that so much did depend on that political struggle. It seemed that hardly anything of importance that happened in society at the time can be explained without reference to it.

The 'compromise' between straight narrative and analysis that could relate to wider questions was greatly helped by the example of one of Kaplan's (1968) largely forgotten works. He built the book around the argument that changes in 1945 should be interpreted as leading to a distinctive 'model' of socialism. He therefore covered the nationalisation of most of industry, changes in social structure, and forms of participation in social life through mass organisations and representative bodies. This was linked to discussion of the programmatic principles of the different political parties, testing which one, or ones, were adequately equipped to help in the development of the emerging, democratic, form of socialism. It was a work that left loose ends, but it seemed an extremely promising starting point.

This I tried to broaden in two directions. One was to cover a longer time span, going back to 1918, to demonstrate a history of continual tensions and evolution in the Communist Party's thinking, and forward through 1948, to show the effects of political dictatorship. The second was to cover a more comprehensive range of changes in economic and political organisation after 1945, rather than nationalisations alone. This, then, was the place for consideration of themes such as the role of factory councils, the position of social groups and the emergence of new organs of power. The discussion of parties' programmes was then developed to show their significance by setting them against the parties' actual behaviour.

Needless to say, none came through with maximum honours. The Communists had shifted markedly from some of their pre-war rhetoric, but had formulated no coherent alternative programme. They still expected a one-party state, but seemed able to achieve many of their social aims without it. There were clearly tensions in their thinking, but arguably no necessity from internal sources for an attempt to seize power. Another striking point to emerge was the relative vacuousness of the thinking on the 'right' of the political spectrum. The National Socialists saw themselves defending pluralist democracy against the threat of totalitarianism. Events in subsequent years would suggest that they should have been wished every success. The trouble was that they had very little more to offer. Their international orientation, hoping for close links with the West but accepting the generally popular orientation towards the East, was undermined with the beginnings of the Cold War. On internal issues they often appeared to be resisting, rather than leading, wider social changes. This gave them a definite social base, but also stimulated animosity and doubts even among some supporters. This was a factor in their inability to mobilise support when it came to the crucial political struggle, a topic covered in later chapters, which concentrated, in a more orthodox way, on deepening divisions leading through the February confrontation.

This broad structure reflects the work's overall argument, incorporated in an obligatory summary of 1400 words in the PhD and in a few paragraphs in the book's introduction. There was, it argued, a possible basis for an alternative to the 'Soviet model', but it depended on further changes in the Communists' thinking. This had been flexible in the past and had undergone changes since the 1930s, so further change was not impossible. Any such prospect was ruled out by the beginnings of the Cold War leading to pressure from the Soviet Union, the exact form of which remained unclear, for the Communists to eliminate opposition and to bring the country firmly into the emerging Soviet bloc. The Communist takeover was widely supported and particularly easy because of the deep and wide-ranging weaknesses identified in other political forces. The establishment of an effective one-party state very quickly demonstrated negative features pointing to still worse times to come.

POINTS OF DETAIL

This general account depended on judgements on points of detail, which had to be confronted with evidence, and decisions taken as to their generalisability, interpretation and significance. This can be illustrated with three examples demonstrating how points of apparent detail interact with overall conclusions.

The first is a dispute that arose around elections to National Committees (the new local government bodies) in early 1946 prior to the parliamentary elections. In a number of cases the National Socialists accused the Communists of intimidating their rivals, thereby supporting claims of imminent totalitarianism and a police state. Their strongest case related to an election in a Prague suburb, where they claimed 20% of the voters had been intimidated into not taking part or, in the case of some Social Democrat supporters, actually imprisoned. This was covered in the competing parties' papers and I concluded that the accusations were unfounded. It was even also possible to check against the parliamentary election results – when there were no accusations of intimidation – which showed the same turnout and a slight swing from the National Socialists to the Communists.

This warranted about a hundred words and reference to five sources in the PhD. It was not mentioned in the book. Had intimidation or ballot rigging been confirmed it would, of course, have been of immense importance. In their absence it could, perhaps, have found a place as a comment on the National Socialists' campaign methods, or the level of their journalism. That might have influenced cooperation between parties, but there was no evidence that it had been important. Even then, it would only have been worth mentioning as an illustration of a general point. In the end, the need for brevity restricted the whole issue to a quote from a National Socialist MP accepting that his party 'did not conduct a clean campaign' (Myant 1981, p. 119). That effectively summarised around one reference the interpretation of a substantial volume of evidence.

This example also illustrates the extent to which readers are expected to trust the author. A large number of newspaper reports led ultimately to a decision to include nothing. Those with practical experience of similar processes of selection and interpretation almost invariably claim that they are being as objective as possible, but the reader is given no explanation or justification for decisions taken. A careless, unscrupulous author, or just one without the background knowledge to spot what is important, could miss the significance of points that 'should' be given prominence, claim unjustified generality for isolated events or select only those examples that fit with a preconceived framework.

The second example illustrates how the quest for a framework can make a 'fact' irresistibly attractive, even when it is 'wrong'. This was an alleged opinion poll in January 1948, which is said to have predicted a drop in the Communist vote in parliamentary elections scheduled for May of that year to 28%. It was reported in a number of works in the West, leading to the assertion that the Communists knew they were losing support and therefore decided to seize power before the elections. It lives on in the textbook by Crampton (1994), who even saw fit to reduce the forecast Communist vote to 25%. He gives no source, but his book generally pays little heed to factual accuracy. Nevertheless, the widespread currency this claim has received would appear to give it some of Carr's characteristics of a 'historical fact'.

The most serious investigation suggests that such a poll was started, but the incomplete returns were never counted (Belda et al. 1968, p. 206). It is impossible to predict accurately what free elections would have yielded, but indicators such as party membership – and by then 40% of the adult population had joined a party – do not point to a dramatic change from 1946. Moreover, there is enough on Communist thinking to leave little doubt that, right up to the February crisis, they rather expected the decisive struggle to come in the elections and expected to find a means to win. They were recognising that they could not achieve this alone, but were cultivating allies in other parties who would later side with them.

Even if there had been serious evidence that such a poll had been conducted, I would have been inclined to dismiss its results as wildly inaccurate, perhaps also casting doubt on the value of other opinion poll results at the time. The Communist leaders at the time might have taken a similar view.

Thus this particular 'historical fact' can be rejected partly because of lack of hard supporting evidence, but partly also because of its incompatibility with related 'facts'. Its popularity stems from the ease with which it seems to support a general account of the period which is oversimplified and hence inaccurate. There is a serious case for ignoring it altogether, a choice that seems to have been taken by Kaplan in a book of about 275 000 words focusing on February 1948 (Kaplan 1996). However, its recurrence in Western sources means that that was not an option for me and the issue is discussed in the book in two paragraphs, with references to three sources.

The third example is the death of Jan Masaryk. The son of Czechoslovakia's first president, T. G. Masaryk, Jan was the non-party Minister for Foreign Affairs from 1945 to 1948. He did not join the ministers who resigned from the government to precipitate the February crisis. His body was found in the courtyard under his flat on the day he was to be included in the new Communist-dominated government. The official verdict was suicide. I accept this as the most likely explanation, with a paragraph's discussion and references to two sources which accepted it as the view of those close to him at the time. To one reviewer this was 'an extraordinary observation' as apparently evidence had come to light that Masaryk was murdered by Soviet agents (Ulč 1982, p. 818). Actually, claims of murder have been based only on rumours and on stories full of assumptions and inaccuracies. As thorough an investigation as is ever likely to be possible, undertaken in 1968–9, led to the conclusion 'that no significant fact has so far emerged that provided evidence for murder' (Kettner & Jedlička 1990, p. 182), while ever more evidence from those close to Masaryk, most notably from his personal secretary (Sum 2003), points very strongly towards suicide. Further determined efforts in the 1990s provided more theories and speculation, but no convincing new evidence. Nevertheless, Ulč's view is so widely accepted that it again fits some of Carr's criteria for consideration as a historical fact.

The issue is both difficult and important. It is difficult because of an established weight of opinion and prejudice that can, as indicated above, use this issue as a major reason for condemning a book. It is important because it can crystallise a number of judgements. It is a single quotable fact that could summarise a more substantial historical investigation and discussion. The alternatives of suicide or murder, presumably involving the Czechoslovak or Soviet security police, have substantial implications for interpretations of the early post-war years. Suicide is consistent with the view that Masaryk felt depressed by events, powerless and maybe ashamed of staying on in the government. He saw no future without close alliance with the USSR – in this he differed from the resigning ministers whose action he felt unable to support – but felt betrayed by the Communists' imposition of a monopoly of power. Suicide fits with a view that his conception of politics had failed and also that he was no threat to anyone. The Communists could have wanted him to stay in office as a cover while they consolidated power. This is the interpretation most consistent with my view of what happened over that period.

Clear evidence of murder would change his standing completely, fitting with a view of a more determined resistance to Communist domination both before and after February 1948. It also fits with a more negative view of the Communist period as a whole, supporting condemnations of brutality from start to finish. It could point to the need for a very substantial reinterpretation of the period, depending on who is found to have killed him.

IS IT ALL SUPERSEDED?

We can conclude around three broad questions relating to whether subsequent work has moved closer to 'objectivity' and 'truth'. The first is to ask whether newly available information would make possible a substantially different kind of work dealing with the period in question. There have been three important advances here. More reflective memoirs have become available, such as the substantial volumes by Prokop Drtina (1982), Minister of Justice from 1945 to 1948. However, he was hampered by political persecution and restricted access to sources, meaning that reflection was limited largely to piecing together the actions of those he had been involved with during the February events.

The second advance has come with access to Czech archival sources, exploited most assiduously by Kaplan, a historian with 88 books to his name in the National Library by 2003, who came to prominence as the main author of the official report on show trials of the early 1950s (Pelikán 1971). He emigrated to Western Germany in 1976, taking notes from researches through official archives. Works after he emigrated to Western Germany in 1976, and back in the Czech Republic after 1989, centre on the 1945–8 period and the early 1950s.

He saw access to archival material as the key to achieving clarity (Kaplan 1996, p. 7) and has provided an enormous amount of new information, for example on how the party leaderships behaved towards each other, on how the police and security forces might have been involved in political conflicts and on how Communist strategy developed. Thus it appears that there were five identifiable, partly overlapping and partly competing, approaches in late 1947 and early 1948. This greater complexity means that, as is familiar in other branches of knowledge, answering some questions does not end the issue, but rather points to further areas for investigation.

The third advance has come with the publication by Russian historians, primarily Galina Murashko, of records from various levels on the Soviet side showing how events in Czechoslovakia were perceived (Prečan et al. 1998; Šiška 1998a, b). They are incomplete and therefore inconclusive, but point to clear Soviet pressure in late 1947 and early 1948 for a speedy resolution of the question of political power and hence for Czechoslovakia's incorporation into the emerging Soviet bloc. Evidence suggests no outright 'orders' from Moscow, but strong implied criticisms of leaving things to be decided by elections and of Gottwald's desire to keep close to constitutional means. There is, however, no support for a view favoured by Kaplan on the basis of one verbal source that the Soviet leadership had been prepared to send troops into the country in February 1948. In fact, Gottwald may have unsuccessfully sought reassurances that a Soviet military intervention was possible, following from fears that substantial internal conflict and disorder might stimulate a US intervention. The Soviet side did not consider this to be a serious possibility.

This fits with my own interpretation of events. It is unfortunate that the amount of information currently available is too limited to allow for certainty.

The second area of questioning relates to whether advances towards the 'truth' have been helped by a new political context, not just in the sense of opening up access to new sources, but rather of leading to the posing of new questions and perhaps to a synthesis overcoming past Cold-War divisions and thinking. This is less clear-cut. A number of new themes have been explored, most notably ones relating to the expulsion of the German minority, which partly reflects a new climate of relations with the reunited Germany. However, although there have since 1989 been no administrative constraints on interpretations of the past, the political climate has encouraged a view of the internal significance of the 1945–8 period largely as the launching pad for Communist rule. Much of the new writing has concentrated on issues of political power and on how the Communists used state organs to their advantage. There has been little original work on other changes in society, on the thinking and lives of the Czech population or on how the period fits into the whole course of Czech history. Ideas of a 'democratic' model of socialism have been of little interest when the dominant rhetoric included a condemnation of socialism of any form.

Kaplan has gone some way in approaching general questions, but there are limits to his archive-based method. He has received some criticism for his own Communist past, as could be expected in post-1989 Czechoslovakia and the Czech Republic. This may have contributed to the cautiousness with which he has made generalisations and gone beyond the safety of points that can be backed up with written sources. It is, for example, remarkable that his massive study of February 1948 contains no discussion of Jan Masaryk's apparent suicide, suggesting that nothing of direct relevance emerged from archival sources he studied.

His main conclusions appear sensible as far as they go, but generally rather modest. The Communists' opponents were, he suggests, bound to lose, but 'they did not need to lose so badly' (1996, p. 539). They failed to understand the nature of their opponent or to see that the struggle would go beyond a standard parliamentary framework. Their 'programmatic inactivity' made it very easy for the Communists, who, as a result, 'did not need to follow the road of a putsch' (p. 539). This amounts to a veiled polemic with President Havel and many others who insisted on using the term 'putsch'. It leaves open questions indicated earlier, relating for example to the parties' programmes and to the apparent paradox that, in contrast to the weaknesses Kaplan identifies, much of their propaganda seemed fixated on warnings of imminent totalitarianism.

The third area of questioning relates to whether my work contributed anything towards a more general advance towards 'truth' and 'objectivity'. It has been referred to and quoted, both negatively and positively, but often for presenting an argument – that there was another possibility ruled out primarily by the international context – that is considered at best unproven. The framework that comes with that, with the space devoted to social and economic changes and to how the thinking of parties related to popular attitudes, probably has influenced and encouraged those who seek to break away from an approach based purely on a fight for political power (e.g. Abrams 2004). In the meantime, the main use of the work has been for the accounts relating to the start of the Cold War or to the Communist takeover, the parts least dependent on original sources. It evidently finds a place as a source judged reasonably objective, written in English and providing 'facts' on themes of some international significance.

ACKNOWLEDGEMENTS

Support from the Carnegie Trust for the Universities of Scotland was used for part of the research on which this contribution is based.

REFERENCES

Abrams, B. (2004) *The Struggle for the Soul of the Nation: Czech Culture and the Rise of Communism*. Rowman & Littlefield, Lanham, MD.

Belda, J., Bouček, M., Deyl, Z., Klimeš, M. (1968) *Na rozhraní dvou epoch*. Svobda, Prague.

Calspace (2002) Climate Change: Past and Future – Discovery of the Great Ice Age, University of California, San Diego. Available at: calspace.ucsd.edu/virtualmuseum/climatechange2/02_1.shtml. Accessed 7 August 2003.

Carr, E. H. (1961) *What Is History?* Penguin, Harmondsworth.

Crampton, R. (1994) *Eastern Europe in the Twentieth Century*. Routledge, London.

Drtina, P. (1982) *Československo můj osud*, 2 vols. Sixty-Eight Publishers, Toronto.

Elton, G. (1967) *The Practice of History*. Sydney University Press, Sydney.

Elton, G. (1991) *Return to Essentials: Some Reflections on the Present State of Historical Study*. Cambridge University Press, Cambridge.

Evans, R. (1997) *In Defence of History*. Granta Books, London.

Hayek, F. (1944) *The Road to Serfdom*. G. Routledge and Sons, London.

Kaplan, K. (1968) *Znárodnění a socialismus*. Academia, Prague.

Kaplan, K. (1996) *Pět kapitol o Únoru*. Doplněk, Brno.

Kettner, P., Jedlička, I. (1990) *Proč zemřel Jan Masaryk?* Horizont, Prague.

Kolb, D. (1984) *Experiential Learning: Experience as the Source of Learning and Development*. Prentice Hall, Englewood Cliffs, NJ.

Kuhn, T. (1962) *The Structure of Scientific Revolutions*. University of Chicago Press, Chicago, IL.

Kuhn, T. (2000) *The Road since Structure: Philosophical Essays, 1970–1993, with an Autobiographical Interview*. University of Chicago Press, Chicago, IL.

Lambert, K., Brittan, G. (1997) *An Introduction to the Philosophy of Science*, 4th edn. Ridgeview, Atascadero, CA.

Marwick, A. (2001) *The New Nature of History: Knowledge, Evidence, Language*. Palgrave, Basingstoke.

Munslow, A. (1997) Reappraisal in history. Available at: www.history.ac.uk/ihr/Focus/What is history/carr1.html. Accessed 20 May 2003.

Myant, M. (1981) *Socialism and Democracy in Czechoslovakia, 1945–1948*. Cambridge University Press, Cambridge.

Pelikán, J. (ed.) (1971) *The Czechoslovak Political Trials 1950–1954: The Suppressed Report of the Dubček Government's Commission of Inquiry, 1968*. Stanford University Press, Stanford, CA.

Popper, K. (1959) *The Logic of Scientific Discovery*. Hutchinson, London.

Popper, K. (1994) *The Myth of the Framework: In Defence of Science and Rationality*. Routledge, London.

Pravda, A. (1982) Driven to dictatorship. *Times Literary Supplement*, 12 March.

Prečan, V., Murašková, G., Gibianskij, L., Kaplan, K. (1998) Zorinova pražská mise v únoru 1948. *Nad novými dokumenty*. Soudobé dějiny, **5**, no. 2–3.

Šiška, M. (1998a) Únor měl předurčeného vítěze. *Právo* 21 February.

Šiška, M. (1998b) Zorinova mise v únoru 1948. *Právo* 28 February.

Sum, A. (ed.) (2003) *Otec a syn II. svazek syn Jan*. Pragma, Prague.

Ulč, O. (1982) Review of Myant, 1981. *American Historical Review*, June.

White, H. (1973) *Metahistory: The Historical Imagination in Nineteenth-Century Europe*. Johns Hopkins University Press, Baltimore, MD.

8 'Scientificity' and its Alternatives: Aspects of Philosophy and Methodology within Media and Cultural Studies Research

NEIL BLAIN

School of Media, Language and Music, University of Paisley, UK

SOME THEORY

The growth of media studies, cultural studies, communication studies and film studies, and their interactions among themselves and with adjacent disciplines, presents too complex a picture to attempt to outline here. They are individually and collectively challenging examples of the notion of academic 'discipline', tending as they do to produce a certain lack of boundedness (a theme further discussed in the next section).

One of their formative practices in the United Kingdom from the 1960s was the exercise of a critique of social and cultural processes, based on a body of thought associated with political economy. A range of writers, some of whose work preceded the foundation of media and cultural studies, produced writing about media, communications and culture which explicitly offered a critique of contemporary social, political and cultural practices.

These writers include Richard Hoggart (1958), Raymond Williams (1962) and Stuart Hall (1958, 1968). Their work is 'critical research', explicitly dissatisfied with a variety of social, political, cultural and above all economic arrangements. In the instance of Williams and Hall, as with many writers toward the beginning of this tradition, it displays a relationship with a variety of Marxist, neo-Marxist or Gramscian stances, modified and enriched over time as their work progresses. The French Marxist philosopher Louis Althusser became a significant influence on anglophone social and cultural critique as his writing was exported, especially his work on the concept of 'ideological state apparatuses' (Althusser 1971).

A philosophically yet more radical stance toward society and culture had developed during the 1960s in the French academy; though in a sense

Interdisciplinary Research: Diverse Approaches in Science, Technology, Health and Society.
Edited by J. Atkinson and M. Crowe.
Copyright © 2006 by John Wiley & Sons, Ltd.

paradoxically, this occurred as at least a partial supercession of Marxist theory. This radical critique produced – to use an adjective most strongly associated with the writing of Jacques Derrida – a *deconstructive* approach to knowledge-gathering, to epistemology and to academic discipline (Derrida 1973, 1976, 1978).

The poststructuralists had a delayed influence on anglophone writing about media and culture, much of which has continued unsusceptible to French influences until the present. But the effect was strong in places. One jibe thrown at the French poststructuralists by English commentators was precisely that they were disappointed Marxist disciples, led to extreme philosophical posturing by the theoretical failures of political economy. (There were other more specific rejections rooted in the tribalism of academic life. When in 1992 Derrida was nominated for an honorary doctorate at Cambridge University a number of academics, including the logician W. V. Quine, signed a letter of objection.) Despite this resistance the longer-term influence of poststructuralism on writing on media and cultural studies in the UK, and particularly in the United States, has been considerable.

Poststructuralism questions the status of all knowledge on the justification that 'knowledge' is produced by language and therefore is variously (depending on the argument) influenced, constrained or falsified by language. In the prior and influential work of both Marx and Nietzsche, 'knowledge' is in any case always offered in the interests of one individual or social group, often against the interests of another. Knowledge, in the Nietzschean perspective, is best understood as power (Norris 1987).

'Poststructuralism', the term generally used to characterise the writing of Derrida and contemporaries such as Michel Foucault, is defined both as issuing from, but greatly modifying, its predecessor, 'structuralism' (Foucault 1975, 1976, 1977).

(Let us remember a 'translation lag', too, which delays the transition of these ideas into anglophone culture by several years – much of Foucault's francophone output is from the 1960s.)

The preceding structuralist tendency in socio-cultural analysis is most strongly associated with the work of Claude Lévi-Strauss, who developed the ideas of the Swiss linguist Ferdinand de Saussure (de Saussure 1974) in order to produce a model of cultural development based on linguistic practice.

(Addressed below, is the further influence on media and cultural studies research of de Saussure in his guise as co-founder of the discipline of semiology, or in its anglophone version, 'semiotics'.)

'Structuralism' in the work of Lévi-Strauss (Lévi-Strauss 1963; Hawkes 1977), and in the writing of those who followed his lead in critical work on cinema of the late 1960s and early 1970s (e.g. Wollen 1969) is precisely that which its offspring 'poststructuralism' would see as a 'grand narrative', in other words, the offer of a totalising theory of the sort which the nineteenth century proposed in the models of Darwin, Freud and Marx. Structuralism offers to explain the world by proposing humankind as a linguistic phenomenon, much as Marxism proposes it as an economic phenomenon, which in Freud or Darwin becomes 'biological'.

'Poststructuralism', which is a philosophical parent of postmodernism theory, retains structuralism's focus on language as the primary human phenomenon, but then inverts it. A general drive in the social sciences toward 'scientificity' is at the heart of Lévi-Strauss's work on the cultures that he investigates. In popular parlance, Lévi-Strauss's structural anthropology can be construed as aiming at the 'harder' rather than the 'softer' end of the social sciences. When Lévi-Strauss writes about the binary functioning of the human brain, he does not intend to be metaphorical. His work on culture is much based upon binary distinctions, most famously between the raw and the cooked. Again, he explains certain aversions, such as a fear of snakes or rats, in terms of our inability to fit these animals into a suitable binary composite – for example, the snake neither swims nor walks, and the rat is neither domestic nor feral.

When discussing what is 'scientific' about such assertions, we revisit different but parallel debates about the work of psychoanalysis, most notably of Freud. We might note here that the subject matter of Freud's work, or Jung's, or that of Lévi-Strauss, is highly complex. Were we speaking of orders of complexity, the study of psychological or cultural drivers would be immensely complex when compared to the study of, for example, single-cell organisms.

Yet structuralism's awkward and brilliant teenager, poststructuralism, eventually grows in its most extravagant moods to question the status of all knowledge (even, by implication, knowledge about single-cell organisms). If knowledge is based on language, and language is both a system of representation and also the medium in which the world is understood, then all knowledge is contingent on language. Moreover, if all knowledge is in Nietzsche's sense 'interested', then we ought with double vigour to contest grand narratives, epistemologies, philosophical and theistic systems; and, of course, academic disciplines.

The linguistic basis of epistemologies is precisely what in the poststructuralist view undermines the claims of disciplines to shape knowledge. In the work of Foucault, 'discipline' becomes a negative term in knowledge (Foucault 1977) associated not with the advance of specific epistemologies but with the narrow interests of the academy and the power struggles of professions such as medicine and law.

Foucault's self-chosen professorial title at the Collège de France, professor of 'the History of Systems of Thought', precisely expresses the possibility that the knowledge to which the academy can lay claim is only the *process of claiming knowledge*. Foucault applies the term 'archaeology' not to 'knowing' something about the past, but to deconstructing the processes of knowledge. This 'deconstructive' trajectory was to invite the hostile accusation that it denied the very possibility of knowledge, though the riposte – that such a process improves knowledge by unmasking false assumptions and claims – is harder to attack.

Foucault's solution for the reconstitution of knowledge was, to put it very simply, to start small, by eschewing large claims and avoiding totalising models. His own work on the French penal system provides a practical example, not least when placed beside his campaigning involvement on prison issues. It has to be said, however, that his view of language as a sort of imprisoning process may itself – contradictorily – be a 'grand narrative'. Nor does his model of knowledge-gathering suggest an escape hatch. How can you get out of the 'prison house' of language (Jameson 1972)?

(But then again, say critics, didn't Foucault himself manage rather well?)

BABEL IN RESEARCH MODE: THE MEDIA AND CULTURAL STUDIES COLLECTIVE

Let us take it for granted that this particular set of French influences nowadays appears in all sorts of disciplines. It certainly provides a context for much media and cultural studies research. Yet very large quantities of research into the media and culture are dismissive or innocent of poststructuralist and postmodernism theory.

Other bodies of theory – quite a few – make themselves known within media and cultural studies. Particularly influential in film studies, for example, is Freudian psychoanalytic theory. Against objections that Freud's 'scientific' status was exploded in the field of psychology many years ago; that Freud is only one of many alternative psychoanalytic theorists (in fact there is also a Jungian film studies field); or that psychoanalysis has been greatly privileged by film theorists over other psychological approaches, Freudian theory still underpins much research into cinema. This phenomenon has been explained unsympathetically, though positive explanations, associated with similarities of the cinematic experience and mental process, including dreams, also offer themselves (for a relatively recent continuance of the Freudian 'scientific' controversy, see for example the debate between Borch-Jacobsen 2000, and Snelling 2001).

A notably awkward aspect of media and cultural studies is that they insist on dragging in other disciplines, and indeed at the core of the definition of media and cultural studies is the notion of *hybridity*. Economics, linguistics, semiotics, sociology, history, politics, psychology, legal studies and nowadays information and computing technology can all be pulled in to play, and often are. There has been a proliferation of related fields such as gender studies.

Alongside theory-driven, anguished researchers questioning the construction of their own identities, are avid historians searching archives for answers; legal experts working on ownership regulations; cultural geographers tracking local media control and influence; linguistic researchers auditing the fate of the adverb in news broadcasts; and gender or ethnicity sociologists counting the number of men or women, or black people, or Muslims, working for the BBC or CNN. These activities all offer their own theoretical contexts, of course, but by no means elevate 'theory' to the heights at which some researchers have placed it in their priorities.

In much research into the domain of media effects, for example, knowledge is still just knowledge. 'The debate is over', declares the American Psychiatric Association, in its public information website section, noting that the 'one overriding finding in research on the mass media is that exposure to media portrayals of violence increases aggressive behavior in children' (Psychiatric Effects of Media Violence, http://www.healthyminds.org/mediaviolence.cfm). It records that the American Academy of Pediatrics recommends that children be exposed at most to one or two hours of television-viewing a day and advocates that exposure to the media in general should be limited.

The writers of these statements know perfectly well that debate about media impacts has been intense and often fevered, research studies presenting a very complex picture, many results evincing little evidence of simple cause-and-effect media impacts. This has been apparent for more than twenty years (McGuire 1986; Gauntlett 1995, 1998; Corner 2000; Cumberbatch 2002). Many researchers have largely abandoned the goal of identifying a simple and determinate link between media messages and human thought or action. But a negative concept of media influence still flourishes in the pronouncements of a variety of researchers and gatekeepers.

Looked at more widely across the academic spectrum, this entirely evident plurality of 'truths' is what has led to the development of 'histories'; for example, in the United States, of alternative black, Hispanic or female histories ('herstories'). The 'textualisation' of history is precisely figured in post-structuralist thought. What can history be if not 'text'? As early as 1957 (in the French original), Roland Barthes posited our understanding of culture as a series of little (or larger) 'myths' (Barthes 1972).

But of course one fierce objection to this trajectory of thought has been political (Norris 1990). We need to know whether the media have effects on children or not. We need to know if we're getting a true picture of the West's various impacts on the Middle East or not. We need to know if historical events are true or not. The validity of Rorty's view to the effect that we can have a civilised debate over such matters (Rorty 1989) seems inadequate, not just because it often isn't enough to have a debate, but also because often our respondents have no wish to debate. Those who declare that the Holocaust was a fiction are not inclined to debate. Those who perpetrated it were not inclined to debate either.

When Jean Baudrillard wrote his celebrated piece in *Libération* to the effect that the first Gulf War had not taken place (Baudrillard 1991) it was intended, ultimately, to stress the extent of the loss of our grasp upon reality, because of the centrality of the media in our lives. He meant: 'what you have witnessed was a media event'. But the piece had great potential to offend. Many people had died, more than have been counted, and to ironise on such a subject was of mixed benefit, particularly in the post-Gulf War 2 perspective now available.

AN AUTOBIOGRAPHICAL REPORT

If all knowledge is 'interested', then that will probably apply to the account so far. This writer has an abiding interest in theory and is well disposed to the poststructuralist inheritance. That is why he – why I, really – begin(s) this piece with an account of Gramscian and poststructuralist approaches to media and cultural studies, rather than, say, with an account of some very fine traditions of film and cinema history.

If I now move to the first person for a while – self-reflexivity has been fashionable in the social sciences for years now – I can report that like many researchers in the media field, I moved from somewhere else, in my case from English literature. (There was not much of a media field to move to when I began teaching in the mid-1970s.) I had written my PhD on the work of the novelist Henry James. It was a traditional literature PhD proposing 'textual expertise' as practised most influentially by F. R. Leavis, whose impact on English studies is still felt. Textual expertise – the professional practice of literary criticism – is a skill, in this perspective, like dentistry. I probably believe that I possess this skill. I suppose that I would otherwise wonder what I was doing for about seven years as an undergraduate and postgraduate student.

This ease with texts which I (think I) developed was the bridge, slightly later in my career, to teaching film, from which I departed to other shores with the confidence typical of a certain kind of literature graduate, who believes that other subjects can thenceforth be colonised at will. This muscular approach with other disciplines is quite typical of media and cultural studies people, who sometimes also shift identities between 'soft' and 'hard' research roles, and between arts-and-humanities and social sciences affiliations.

In fact, media and cultural studies research tasks often require a broad education in the researcher. Sociologists, for example, who study the media (becoming 'media sociologists') frequently do not handle texts well, or sufficiently. Another example: a lack of philosophical background will and does hamper many kinds of researchers trying to come to terms with theoretical problems in culture. Again: the development of what is referred to either as 'semiology' or 'semiotics', broadly, the 'science of signs', has produced an often highly specialised body of concepts, terminology and theory dependent on a degree of familiarity with other disciplines (for example, philosophy and linguistics). It is *semiotics* which one often encounters early on as a term in the debate within media and cultural studies about quantitative, qualitative and theoretical dimensions of the field, not least in relation to the inadequacies of 'content analysis'.

My own work has encompassed theoretical development of arguments about collective identity and symbolic process (e.g. about sport as a symbolic process), and also historical research, say, into the history of Scottish documentary film, and textual work on media constructions of social and cultural process, especially into 'European identities' and the media. But despite my louche (though admittedly distant) background in English and American literature, I have also conducted 'hard', quantitative research, for example as a consultant for the broadcasting industry. I developed this largely through being 'apprenticed' to people working in the market research industry. I have therefore had to justify the expenditure of substantial sums of money to very shrewd broadcasting managers suffering from consultant fatigue. This gives me a particular perspective on my other interests, for example in postmodernism theory.

When I lecture to students on research methods, and when I try to deal with the theoretical dimensions of contemporary approaches to epistemology, I point out to them that the poststructuralist approach is appropriate in its context, but can easily be misplaced. Let us take, for example, Baudrillard's contention that the nineteenth-century concept of ideology is not up to the task of explaining the symbolic workings of the media age. Baudrillard notes that the concept of ideology in Marx's sense 'masks and perverts a basic reality'. This is what Baudrillard, speaking historically, calls 'the second phase of the image' – its first, of course, is that it just represents something, fair and simple. But in the media age, he continues, the predominance of 'representation' over 'substance' means that the original real-world 'object' or 'event' being represented becomes overwhelmed by the processes of representation. This is the 'third phase of the image', in which signs (e.g. television programmes) mask 'the absence of a basic reality' (Baudrillard 1983).

The idea that 'reality had disappeared' when Baudrillard wrote this in the last quarter of the twentieth century, was – in the age of the *National Enquirer*, and many a successful historical hoax – not necessarily startling. It is actually quite a useful idea, theoretically.

If, on the other hand, you are presenting research results, as I have, to a couple of dozen senior television managers, many thousands of pounds of whose funds you have just been spending, it is not advisable to preface your comments by noting that your findings and conclusions mask a basic absence of reality. I have not tried this, and I would not recommend it.

Of course, the appropriateness of such a preamble would depend on what you were trying to find out. If I am giving students a good example of a reliable association between representation and reality, I will choose a case where I am driving on the M6 motorway and a radio announcer tells me there is a serious traffic delay ahead. I look in vain for an exit road, and encounter the blockage, in which I sit for the next ninety minutes. This is the 'first phase of the image', pure and simple. Something is represented as true and it is true. This happens all the time. It is the basis of social and cultural organisation. Without this sort of reliability human society could not have developed. Signs, including market research, often very accurately represent the real world. Experts on econometrics in advertising are with great frequency proven to be correct in their representation of social structure, attitude and consumer behaviour.

As far as audience research is concerned: if I have to find out how many television viewers either have, or are planning soon to have, digital satellite capacity in their houses, I know how to do that. If you want a reliable result, you have to subcontract a market research company big enough to access a large stratified sample of the population, and if you need yet more data of this kind at the same time – how do people feel about satellite versus cable provision? – then you may have to pay informants for visits to their houses by fieldworkers, which will have to be in many different locations. This is expensive but fairly reliable if done properly.

However, if you want to find out if British people would like more regional television programming, the whole business gets more complex. If you ask informants if (say) they would like more features on the countryside or town where they live, they may just say 'yes', but the question if casually constructed will have the same effect as asking 'would you like a nice cup of tea and a biscuit?': in other words, you will not really know what they mean by 'yes'. Which of these is it: 'yes, *I really do want that so much that it would influence my channel loyalty*'; or 'yes, *I want that just marginally more than I don't, and yes is nicer than saying no*'; or 'yes, *I'm just saying "yes" at random, really*'?

Since you can't reasonably spend money to get vague results like that, you work away at the questions to minimise the scope for misinterpretation. But some 'realities' are much easier to 'represent' than others.

Of course, that's just the beginning of the difficulties, because sometimes if clients for a research project like the sound of a response from a focus group, they might wish to act upon some aberrant declaration from an informant, even if you would have needed twelve hundred and not twelve informants in the sample to determine its value. So, ironically, you can easily end up asking clients not to take some of your findings too seriously: this here is 'reliable' but that there is just 'indicative'. I once, many years ago, walked into a broadcasting headquarters the morning after a very famous consultant's report had been published and was on every news broadcast; much debate hinging on its findings. I mentioned it to a senior manager of the organisation that had spent much money on its commission. He looked at me disbelievingly. 'Are you kidding? That's a load of crap,' he said, 'we're not paying *any* attention to that *what-so-ever*', spelling out the last four syllables contemptuously.

In the next section, I reproduce some of my own earlier writing in a self-critical spirit. My previous work for broadcasters has been entirely protected from discussion by commercial confidentiality, and is therefore not under further consideration here. After hearing the response reported above, nor did I ever go out of my way to seek feedback from them, beyond what was necessary.

THE PROBLEM OF CULTURE (I): BIG ASSERTIONS

Evidently what follows will traverse only a part of the landscape outlined above. The emphasis hereafter will be on questions that in a broad way try to illustrate some methodological issues in writing about culture. My subject here is (of all things) monarchy. In 2003 I brought out a book with my co-author Hugh O'Donnell on the topic. Greatly simplified, the central thesis of the book is that the British monarchy and royal family operate symbolically to strengthen a British identity which is largely backward-looking and conservative, as distinct from their European equivalents, constructed in the European media as providing evidence of the political modernity of European states. The book is critical of the British media obsession with royalty and pessimistic about the effects of such constructed importance, which are posited as politically significant, and largely negative. Conclusions are also drawn about Britain's relationship with Europe, and vice versa, and about the nature of any possible British republicanism.

The book draws, among other sources, on earlier work on the British monarchy and royal families by Tom Nairn (1988) and also Michael Billig (1992) but in much larger part focuses on a development of cultural theory to provide an explanation of differences in the symbolic functioning of monarchy across Europe, all the while grounding the theoretical work in very large quantities of textual example from the media of the five central countries. There is some further material, for example from Sweden, and – beyond either Europe or monarchy – the United States. The book focuses (for reasons detailed therein) particularly on the Spanish, Dutch, Belgian and Norwegian monarchies and royal families alongside those of the United Kingdom.

The authors were well aware in advance that a project of this sort was not only very difficult but that such an undertaking raised objections from other researchers that it was not possible to engage in useful comparison on this scale, and for a variety of reasons; for example because conclusions drawn might be superficial or mistaken. But the book emerged from a series of comparative writings during the 1990s which were quite consciously based on an opposing view, namely that much writing on issues of ideology and power which emerged from media and cultural studies, from linguistics, and from elsewhere in the social sciences, was hampered by lack of theoretical scale and connection, and was negatively rather than positively constrained by discipline boundedness.

The prototype piece for a theorised cross-European project was a plenary paper delivered by the authors at the University of Pamplona and subsequently published (Blain & O'Donnell 1991). In the wake of the publication (with a third author, Raymond Boyle) of *Sport and National Identity in the European Media* (Blain et al. 1993), both authors had intermittently addressed these themes for a further decade (e.g. O'Donnell 1994; Blain & O'Donnell 1998; Bernstein & Blain 2002) while pursuing other research. *Sport and National Identity in the European Media* had also been acknowledged internationally as an influence on a number of subsequent studies and the authors of the monarchy book did not enter the project defensively, its methodology by now having a long history.

With that distinction in mind which was made above about Foucault's trajectory, i.e. between 'small', more easily established assertions about culture, and larger 'totalising' assertions, the monarchy book covers a significant part of the spectrum from the analysis of small cultural phenomena to rather large phenomena. For example, its lengthy concluding section makes some assertions about differences between Britain and Europe, which are on the face of things very risky.

Here is the opening paragraph of the Conclusion. The first sentence is possibly the punchline of the book, or would be, were it reducible to one, which its authors rather hope it isn't:

Political modernity
The most striking fact among many comparative features of European monarchy, as we noted in the Introduction, is that Britain's is the only monarchy not required to justify itself by its contribution to political modernity. The other monarchies we have been studying here are clearly constructed in the public sphere as maintaining or augmenting or, as in the Spanish case, inaugurating and even saving, conditions of political modernity. In an ambivalent instance, in The Netherlands, the media are strongly sensitive about any impediment the performance and symbolism of the House of Orange presents to Dutch political modernity. As was seen earlier, the Spanish monarchy in relation to modernity has virtually a reverse symbolic function from the UK's. In Spain, when democracy was threatened by coup, 'the King was in his place, defending democracy when he needed to' (*El País*, 22 November 2000). Spain was in a sense inoculated against the postmodernization of its politics by General Franco, and there is little sign of the dosage wearing off, despite changes to other aspects of Spanish culture. When democracy can still be felt as an acquisition which needs to be defended, monarchy is much more likely to remain politicized than become postmodernized.

I begin with this, because it provides a context for what follows. Since to pursue every methodological argument arising out of even this brief set of statements would imply a lengthy process of argumentation, it is better to concentrate on some central questions.

Is the purpose of a Conclusion which begins in this manner to furnish objective proof of cultural and political phenomena? Probably among the ripostes to that – were it an assertion rather than a question – would be: 'it is inconceivable that such an assertion can be sustained because of all the questions and doubts it invites'. For example, in the first sentence, I write that 'Britain's is the only monarchy not required to justify itself by its contribution to political modernity'. An obvious question is: 'not required by whom – did you interview a representative sample of informants in Britain, and ask them?'

'No,' I reply, 'this book's main empirical evidence is media content'.

'What does that prove?'

Well, even at this elementary stage, we are in the presence of quite a debate.

As mentioned, *Sport and National Identity in the European Media* (Blain et al. 1993) used media contents to raise questions about national and transnational identity. There, we advanced some justifications for using media contents as a form of evidence about social and cultural characteristics. We also cited the vast quantity of media texts which we analysed. But even at that time – when, simultaneously and with a rather different research persona I was doing quantitative work for the broadcasting industry – the 'quantitative' dimension of the sport research was something we conceived of as a sort of necessary gesture to a particular concept of verification. That isn't to say that the numbers weren't important (we cited 3 000 reports) but that we might have comfortably lived with fewer, and produced the same conclusions.

There lies a further complication. Does research on complex cultural themes primarily assert objectively verifiable evidence, seek to promote argument or (as in the view of Nietzsche and Foucault) advance causes? When I have taught courses on complex subjects such as cultural theory, I have often found myself saying to students that the quality of their questions in written work is much more significant than their answers. This is because we are in either explicit or tacit agreement to the effect that these themes are too complex for us to conceive of definitive answers to the questions they raise.

An example: there have been some fairly extravagant claims over recent years about the nature of something called 'the postmodern self', often conceived of as a 'consumption-orientated self', by which people achieve definition through acts of consumption and 'empowerment' at moments of transaction (in stores or on Internet retail sites). I used to ask students on my Cultural Theory course in a previous university a question at the beginning of the semester, which I wanted them to answer by the end, namely: 'what are you, that is, what is your identity, what constitutes *yourself*, which is *not* implicated in the process of consumption?'. I gave them most of the semester to think about this and then we had a couple of theory-based seminars on it at the end. These were usually quite good fun and I hope fairly valuable but no one thought for a moment that we could answer questions like this, e.g. that we could conceive of any metrics which might be applicable to the question.

Of course we might have made a start, breaking the waking hours into different kinds of acts, and building a taxonomy of self-statements, but even to define 'consumption' becomes very difficult in an age of 'postmodern ethics', in which even 'ethical' labour can be read as 'self-branding'. I got some nice simple answers from students ('I help out at a swimming group' was one which defied the groups' attempts to turn it into an act of consumption, though no doubt it could have been): but no one started the process by conceiving of the possibility of an objective resolution of the question. (Perhaps the idea of the 'consumer self' is really a metaphor, and belongs to the domain of art: to that idea I return in the conclusion.)

So that – returning to the opening quotation from the monarchy book – the context in which we read cultural research is not necessarily the context in which we read other kinds of research.

Of course if I repeat a sentence from a few paragraphs above:

Does research on complex cultural themes primarily assert objectively verifiable evidence, or seek to promote argument or advance causes?

it should be clear that it might also apply to every conceivable field of research from economics to small-particle physics. I will not reopen here familiar arguments about *inductive* and *deductive* approaches to the real world but there are elements of the debate on cultural research which differ little from debate on any field of research in which people make assertions, or practise belief.

Conversely: if verifiable evidence conforms, as one of its tests, to the capacity accurately to predict recurring or future phenomena, then our work on sport and identity in Europe did that quite well in 1993, making some predictions about aspects of European culture which proved to be very accurate.

Yet when it comes (for example) to making assertions of the kind which we offer in our monarchy book, for example, that we believe that European societies have postmodernised at different rates, we make a claim which must by its nature be contested. A paragraph such as this one:

Let us finally again note that the structure within which the (predominantly) UK-focused royal examples above are understood, that is, in relation to the categories of the modern and the postmodern, holds good for the UK. In Spain, Norway, Belgium and The Netherlands, we gather local evidence for different patterns of development, analyzed in the central section below.

might even at the most fundamental level be challenged, namely, on the grounds that many researchers and writers working on themes of contemporary society, politics and culture do not use the latter category of the 'postmodern' at all. Given that the academic community cannot even agree on the existence of the phenomenon of 'postmodernity', how is it possible to assert that countries can have postmodernised at different rates? Put another way, what kind of 'truth claim' is this?

As always, there is a set of answers to this, too, for example, that the idea of 'uneven development' has long been a staple of discussion about modernity. Since many of us cannot conceive of contemporary European development without the category of the postmodern, it would also be quite unreasonable to assume that Europe could postmodernise evenly, and we think it would be naïve and even aberrant of us to suggest anything else. Of course, in the book,

and because we cannot 'prove' the postmodernisation of Europe or its uneven-
ness, we cite other writers and researchers who support our case. In turn we
have done that because we believe the case is just.

A major source of this belief, underpinning our book, is a domain which
many of us with arts backgrounds are at home in: the domain of the *textual*.

THE PROBLEM OF CULTURE (II): SMALL ASSERTIONS

For example, we research huge quantities (yes – quantitativeness again!) of
media output on monarchy and we find references to 'Big Brother with a
family tree' (Dutch *NRC Handelsblad* on the Dutch monarchy, 16 May 2001);
or Norway's *Dagbladet*, on their prince's relationship with a single working
mother with an interesting past as constituting:

> the beginning of a comprehensive modernisation of the monarchy where open-
> ness, closeness to the people and a strong social commitment are important ele-
> ments. But it can also be the beginning of the end because the throne is
> increasingly experienced as a piece of furniture from IKEA.
>
> (15 April 2000)

Helpfully, the same newspaper runs an editorial the next month entitled 'Postmodern monarchy'. With this and other evidence we become adventurous:

> We analyze in Chapter 7 an extraordinary article on the Norwegian engagement
> which explicitly constructs the imminent royal wedding as part of a consumer and
> media landscape from which it is indistinguishable, like fact and fiction themselves.
> As Norwegian society *postmodernizes* there are increasing calls from broadly left-
> wing sources for a *modernization* of the monarchy.

'Triangulation' might seem an unusual concept to introduce here but it isn't
really, even in this context. Most interpretations of cultural phenomena follow
a process of dialogue between data and theorisation, and that process of dialogue includes one's own data and theorisation, and other people's data and
theorisation. In this instance the authors of this monarchy book have spent 15
years intermittently writing about trans-European cultural questions within
what is effectively – and often actively – a community of researchers whose
ideas develop in juxtaposition with each other's data and theoretical arguments, and which constantly test themselves against cultural evidence.

This length of time is, for example, long enough to determine whether other
academics think one's ideas are aberrant or useful. I cannot recall any of these
broad assertions about European culture being contested on methodological
grounds, odd as that may seem in such perilous territory, though this work has
often been engaged.

And what may seem like stretching the 'triangulation' case, but isn't – at
least I don't think so – in the cultural domain: I have also discussed cultural
and political matters a great deal in public forums including broadcast media,

and because these discussions have often implicated my academic interests, I've received some useful 'reality checks' from outside the academic community. It is very important to say this. I am sceptical of claims to truth about culture and society which are tested by debate only within academic communities. Many other kinds of claims can of course be tested only there, because of the specialised nature of the data and the theory, but where I am clearest in my direction as a researcher is where I've had to defend broad cultural assertions to a demographic variety of audiences (and, of course, internationally).

However, there is also the suggestion so far that (in our monarchy research) 'the text' has some special status.

The last and rather more extended example from our book is a 'textual' analysis which in my case brings my original English Studies persona together with a current professional identity within the species 'cultural theorist'.

This extract is about the funeral of Princess Diana. As elsewhere in the book, the account combines theoretical accounts with the empirical data; for example, we suggest that Diana as a socio-cultural and economic phenomenon is produced by a list of factors centrally including:

- the post-1973 phase of what Harvey (1989) refers to as 'flexible accumulation';
- a high degree of mediatisation, including development of new technologies;
- a loss of public subscription to representative forms of democracy;
- globalisation;
- diminution of the high/low culture divide (aspect of 'aestheticisation' of culture);
- cult of celebrity (a further aesthetic feature);
- entrepreneurialism in sentimental realm;
- 'Latinisation' of British culture (patterns of grieving post-Heysel, Hillsborough, perhaps as sub-feature of globalisation).

The box presents a textual analysis of a small part of the BBC's account of the funeral.

Box 8.1. BBC: eve of funeral; morning of funeral

On the eve of the funeral, *Diana, the People's Vigil* was presented on BBC by one of the channel's heavyweight presenters, David Dimbleby. It begins with a zoom out from the tower of Big Ben against a black sky: 'Big Ben in London telling us that it's just after half-past ten: and the thoughts of the whole country are turning towards this part of the city, to Westminster Abbey, whose west front is floodlit tonight . . .'.

After a short introductory sequence, there follows a montage of a dozen slow motion soft-edged shots of Diana as mother; helper of the aged; with the sick; with Mother Theresa of Calcutta; punctuated here and there by shots of lilies, accompanied by a nostalgic popular piano track. This sequence ends with the title *Diana, the Nation's Vigil*, over a complex montage comprising a still of a serious-looking Diana to the left, with a shot of a bunch of lilies framing the right, in motion, over an abstract background, the latter shot dissolving into a live shot of the crowd (an intriguing editorial confection). After a further address from Dimbleby, of a nationally-unifying character, the reporter addresses the camera from the Mall.

Reporter 1: 'Well this is the scene in the Mall this evening, already hundreds of people lining the route prepared for a damp, possibly showery night, so that they can pay their respects tomorrow to Diana Princess of Wales. People have been coming from all over the country to really . . . be a symbol of a United Kingdom, a kingdom it seems already so united in grief. People have all their own memories of Diana, they want to share them with other people, they talk about her constantly, they also are rather shocked and still have a lot of disbelief that such a young woman, such a vibrant, caring young woman has had her life cut so tragically short . . .' (this already presents a complex mixture of reporting and editorializing; as will be seen, we surmise that the reporter is uncomfortable at having to overrule a professional instinct merely to report – whereas the staging demands a clearly themed narrative) (Blain & O'Donnell 2003).

At this point the reporter turns to her left, taking a pace or so backwards, to an obviously prepared vox pop: 'A family here, just behind me, they're already bedded down for this evening – can you tell me why you're prepared to stay the night here?', bending down to a young woman accompanied by two children in sleeping bags. 'It's just something I've got to do, just got to be here, pay my respects to Diana, she was, she's just, nobody will ever replace her, nobody could try, (I) mean we've just got to be here, it's the last thing, the only thing we can do.' This is delivered calmly and evenly, after which the reporter steps towards the young boys in the sleeping bags with 'And these are your sons down here, are they?' 'Yes they are.' 'What did Diana mean to you?' The boys deliver themselves politely and cheerfully, and with evident relief, of prepared statements. The younger says 'She was kind and she did a lot for other people' and then turns to his elder brother on cue, as does the reporter, and he says, 'She was a very special lady'. His younger brother grins with relief as the second response is given.

At its most plausible this interview is a mixture of what is no doubt a genuine enough response by the mother (though we cannot know this) and what seems like a piece of television rhetoric involving the children. This becomes yet clearer in the next phase of the interview. Continuing to address the elder, the reporter asks: 'Have you ever done anything like this before, camped out in the freezing cold?' 'No', he replies, as does his brother. 'Do you think you'd do it for anyone else?' the reporter asks the elder. 'Probably not', he replies, and the younger shakes his head with a smile which plainly says that he wasn't warned about this extension of the discussion, indicating that the interview has already exceeded its expected demands – the boys are plainly keen to acquit themselves well, and don't want to get involved in any more extemporized utterances. 'Well,' says the reporter, standing up after a half-pause and moving off with a smile, 'some emotions there from two very young lads. And something of course that they'll remember for the rest of their lives as well'. It has to be said that there have been no emotions, as such, visible at all from either of the boys, who simply appear well brought up and anxious to complete a demanding task properly. But British television journalists have been well schooled to seek the emotional response as the *sine qua non* of any likely exchange, no matter how brief ('can you tell us how you feel?').

As for memories: Michael Billig's invaluable social psychological study (based on interviews conducted in late 1988 and throughout 1989 with families talking about the British royals) in one instance records a royalist mother trying to get her sceptical son to admit that he has watched royal weddings. He says he did but that 'I can't remember my feelings at the time, but I remember watching it on tv'. The mother does not really accept that he doesn't remember how he felt:

> Then, she returned to the ceremonies. If Charles were to be crowned king, she said turning to her radical son, wouldn't you feel it was a memorable event, something to tell your grandchildren about? Hang on a minute, he replied, what have you told me about the Coronation of '53? 'We've never had reason to', she answered, 'I mean you've never said "Mum tell us about 1953"'. (Billig 1992, pp. 37–38)

There is an important difference between 'remembering your feelings' and remembering watching something on TV. This exchange shows the son trying to establish the not unreasonable claim that if royal events are really so important and symbolically enduring, then he would have expected to have thought about them a little during his life. Logically, had his mother thought the Coronation of 1953 important, she might previously have mentioned it.

The specifically textual element in the analysis here is placed within a tradition of social and cultural critique mentioned at the start of this essay. Its intention is to question the apparent 'naturalness' of the coverage and to try to make visible the 'constructedness' of the televisual event. Behind that attempt is a sense of the BBC knowingly or unwittingly serving a conservative function. The book is agnostic as to the degree of volition or awareness in this stance by the BBC. The textual analysis here, however, moves beyond description to interpretation.

How can such interpretations be sustained? In practice when writing this account, I am moving back and forth between my prior sense that the BBC does tend to adopt conservative ideological stances in relation to such events, and what I take to be the objective textual evidence on this occasion. That prior sense of the BBC's ideological position has in the first place been derived from my experience of textual characteristics. If that sense is bolstered by accounts from other researchers I begin to feel a sense of confidence that my reading is not aberrant. I also rely here on what I take to be my skill in interpreting verbal and non-verbal signals (well, I've taught sociolinguistics and non-verbal communication, so why not?) as well as on experience in analysing TV material. I then – rhetorically? – appeal to Billig's work to try to establish from a further source that it is possible that royal events are neither as memorable nor as significant as televisual accounts suggest. Is my *intention* to offer a 'critique' a flaw in my objective stance? No. I'm taking issue with the BBC's claim to offer an objective stance. And Billig's findings are based on very sound ethnographic fieldwork; and we cite further solid fieldwork findings from a different researcher later in the book (Turnock 2000).

CONCLUSION

Researching culture, then, is at least as complex as researching very small physical particles and there may be equal quantities of disagreement over their nature.

Are qualities like 'interpretativeness' or 'creativity' more characteristic in the former than the latter domain? It is small-particle physics, after all, which went to James Joyce's greatest novel in order to name sub-atomic 'quarks': and, speaking of physics, the distance between a four-dimensional universe and a universe with dimensions reaching into double figures is grounds for a larger argument than can be held about postmodernity. (Probably.)

Yet where culture is concerned there is indeed an unbroken arc from cultural critique right into the domain of art. I have long taught students on the theme of modernity, and like many others (Berman 1983; Williams 1985) when I want to turn to 'proofs' of modernity I turn first not to scholars but to poets and painters and novelists. It is in Baudelaire and Dostoyevsky that we find the sedimented evidence of the psychological experience of the developed modern city:

> La rue assourdissante autour de moi hurlait.
> Longue, mince, en grand deuil, douleur majestueuse,
> Une femme passa, d'une main fastueuse
> Soulevant, balançant le feston et l'ourlet . . .
>
> Un éclair . . . puis la nuit! – Fugitive beauté
> Dont le regard m'a fait soudainement renaître,
> Ne te verrai-je plus que dans l'éternité?

[The deafening street was screaming all around me.
Tall, slender, in deep mourning – majestic grief –
A woman made her way, with fastidious hand
Raising and swaying festoon and hem . . .

A lightning-flash . . . then night! – O fleeting beauty
Whose glance all of a sudden gave me new birth,
Shall I see you again only in eternity?]
(Baudelaire, extracts from 'A une passante', published in
Les Fleurs du Mal 1857, translated Howard 1982)

Wordsworth, back at the start of the same century (more 'triangulation'!), has seen the same new phenomena in London:

O Friend! one feeling was there which belonged
to this great city, by exclusive right;
How often, in the overflowing streets,
Have I gone forward with the crowd and said
Unto myself, 'The face of every one
That passes by me is a mystery!'
(Prelude VII, Preludes, 1798–1805; see also Williams 1985)

It is the German 'science' of hermeneutics (Bleicher 1980, 1982), too large a topic for this essay, which has come closest to a truly systematic approach to the analysis of culture. Yet even there, the notion of a 'skill' or an 'art' in cultural observation is perfectly consistent with its tenets. What would be the place of 'skill' and 'art' in other disciplines? But perhaps these are enough questions to be going on with.

ACKNOWLEDGEMENTS

I should like to thank Intellect for their kind permission to publish extracts from *Media, Monarchy and Power*; my colleagues Hugh O'Donnell, for his role in the development of the body of writing described here, Rinella Cere and John W. Robertson, for taking the trouble to read an earlier draft of this chapter, and John Atkinson and Malcolm Crowe, for their encouragement.

REFERENCES

Althusser, L. (1971) *Lenin and Philosophy*. New Left Books, London.
Barthes, R. (1972) *Mythologies*. Jonathan Cape, London.
Baudelaire, C. (1982) *Les Fleurs du Mal* (trans. R. Howard). David R. Godine, Boston, MA.
Baudrillard, J. (1983) *Simulacra and Simulations*. Sémiotext(e), New York.
Baudrillard, J. (1991) La guerre du Golfe n'a pas eu lieu. *Libération*, 29 March.
Berman, M. (1983) *All That Is Solid Melts Into Air*. Verso, London.

Bernstein, A., Blain, N. (eds) (2002) *Culture, Sport, Society* **5**(3), Special Edition on Sport and the Media.

Billig, M. (1992, 1998) *Talking of the Royal Family*. Routledge, London.

Blain, N., O'Donnell, H. (1991) Italia 90 en la prensa europea: historias de la vida nacional. In C. Barrera & M. A. Jimeno (eds) *La información como relato* (pp. 15–81). University of Pamplona, Pamplona.

Blain, N., O'Donnell, H. (1998) Living without the *Sun*: European sports journalism and its readers during Euro '96. In M. Roche (ed.) *Sport, Popular Culture and Identity* (pp. 37–56). Meyer and Meyer, Aachen.

Blain, N., O'Donnell, H. (2003) *Media, Monarchy and Power*. Intellect, Bristol.

Blain, N., Boyle, R., O'Donnell, H. (1993) *Sport and National Identity in the European Media*. Leicester University Press, Leicester.

Bleicher, J. (1980) *Contemporary Hermeneutics*. Routledge and Kegan Paul, London.

Bleicher, J. (1982) *The Hermeneutic Imagination*. Routledge and Kegan Paul, London.

Borch-Jacobsen, M. (2000) How a fabrication differs from a lie. *London Review of Books*, 13 April.

Corner, J. (2000) Influence: the contested core of media research. In J. Curran & M. Gurevitch (eds) *Mass Media and Society* (pp. 376–397). Arnold, Oxford.

Cumberbatch, G. (2002) Media effects: the continuing controversy. In A. Briggs & P. Cobley (eds) *The Media: An Introduction* (pp. 259–271). Longman, Harlow.

Derrida, J. (1973) *Speech and Phenomena, and Other Essays on Husserl's Theory of Signs* (trans. David B. Allison). Northwestern University Press, Evanston, IL.

Derrida, J. (1976) *Of Grammatology* (trans. Gayatri Chakravorty Spivak). Johns Hopkins University Press, Baltimore, MD.

Derrida, J. (1978) *Writing and Difference* (trans. Alan Bass). University of Chicago Press, Chicago, IL.

Foucault, M. (1975) *Madness and Civilization: A History of Insanity in the Age of Reason*. Tavistock, London.

Foucault, M. (1976) *The Archaeology of Knowledge*. Harper Colophon, New York.

Foucault, M. (1977) *Discipline and Punish: The Birth of the Prison*. Penguin, Harmondsworth.

Gauntlett, D. (1995) *Moving Experiences: Understanding Television's Influences and Effects*. John Libbey Media, London.

Gauntlett, D. (1998) Ten things wrong with the 'effects model'. In R. Dickinson, R. Harindranath & O. Linné (eds) *Approaches to Audiences – A Reader*. Arnold, London.

Hall, S. (1958) A sense of classlessness. *Universities and Left Review* **1**, 26–32.

Hall, S. (1968) Class and the mass media. In R. Mabey (ed.) *Class: A Symposium*. Blond, London.

Harvey, D. (1989) *The Condition of Postmodernity*. Blackwell, Oxford.

Hawkes, T. (1977) *Structuralism and Semiotics*. Methuen, London.

Hoggart, R. (1958) *The Uses of Literacy*. Penguin, Harmondsworth.

Jameson, F. (1972) *The Prison House of Language*. Princeton University Press, Princeton, NJ.

Lévi-Strauss, C. (1963) *Structural Anthropology*. Basic Books, New York.

McGuire, W. J. (1986) The myth of massive media impact. In G. Comstock (ed.) *Public Communication and Behaviour* (vol. 1). Academic Press, Orlando, FL.

Nairn, T. (1988) *The Enchanted Glass*. Radius, London.

Norris, C. (1987) *Derrida*. Fontana Press, London.

Norris, C. (1990) *What's Wrong with Postmodernism: Critical Theory and the Ends of Philosophy*. Harvester, London.

O'Donnell, H. (1994) Mapping the mythical: a geopolitics of national sporting stereotypes. *Discourse and Society* **5**, 3.

Rorty, R. (1989) *Contingency, Irony and Solidarity*. Cambridge University Press, Cambridge.

de Saussure, F. (1974) *Course in General Linguistics*. Fontana/Collins, Glasgow.

Snelling, D. (2001) In a cool and scientifically objective spirit: perverting reason and truth in the Freud Case. Available at www.psychoanalysis.org.uk/snelling.htm. Accessed January 2006.

Turnock, R. (2000) *Interpreting Diana*. BFI, London.

Williams, R. (1962) *Communications*. Penguin, Harmondsworth.

Williams, R. (1985) The metropolis and the emergence of modernism. In E. Timms & D. Kelley (eds) *Unreal City: Urban Experience in Modern European Literature and Art*. Manchester University Press, Manchester.

Wollen, P. (1969) *Signs and Meaning in the Cinema*. Secker and Warburg/BFI, London.

9 The Truth as Personal Documentation: An Anthropological Narrative of Hospital Portering

NIGEL RAPPORT
Concordia University, Montreal, Canada

INTRODUCTION: QUALITATIVE AND QUANTITATIVE METHODOLOGIES

Disagreements over the nature of qualitative as against quantitative research methodologies interestingly point to a query regarding the nature of the discipline of sociocultural anthropology as such: art or science?[1] When considering the range of methods of gathering data which anthropologists today employ – participant-observation, life-histories, genealogies, censuses, questionnaires, interviews, focus-group discussions, network analysis, archival transcription, video-recording – and the difficulty of deciding whether each is 'qualitative' or 'quantitative', and to what extent, it becomes clear that the latter distinction is more one of overall orientation and intention: 'qualitative' and 'quantitative' as significant emblems.

At the heart of the division is a disagreement over the relationship between anthropological knowledge and the replication of information. For something to be true, does it have to be observably replicated or replicatable (quantitative); and does a sample of events of the same kind have to be taken into account so that the representativeness of the new information can be ascertained? Alternatively, can one accept something is true if observed only by one person on one occasion (qualitative), both the manner of observation and the nature of the thing observed precluding replication; cannot something be imagined to be true if it is unique, its own kind, and while implicated in other things is not them and not like them?

Secondary oppositions then follow in the wake of this question of replication, and extend the division. For instance: is it necessary to explain subjects from an independent, extraneous, purportedly objective standpoint ('quantitative'), or

Interdisciplinary Research: Diverse Approaches in Science, Technology, Health and Society.
Edited by J. Atkinson and M. Crowe.
Copyright © 2006 by John Wiley & Sons, Ltd.

can explanation be subjective, and admit a particular point of view ('qualitative')? Should the researcher begin with a directing hypothesis ('quantitative'), or with an open mind, cleared as far as possible of preconceptions concerning the nature of his research subjects ('qualitative')? Should research identify variables and causal relations, which, it is hoped, possess universal provenance ('quantitative'), or is it sufficient to disinter substantive concepts and theories that are known to be locally grounded ('qualitative')? Should the researcher restrict himself to sensory observation and the control of reason ('quantitative'), or allow himself to empathise, introspect and intuit meanings and relations ('qualitative')?

In part, the opposition between the qualitative and the quantitative can be seen to be an anachronism: a throwback to nineteenth-century conceptions of science, and attempts by social science to ape the reputed certainty of its methods of measurement and so borrow from its legitimacy and status. With the advent of twentieth-century science – Einsteinian relativity, quantum mechanics, chaos theory – comes a new ethos, however: an appreciation of the contingency, situatedness and intrusiveness – alternatively, the creativeness – of the research process as such. Conveniently summed up by 'Heisenberg's uncertainty principle', here is a realisation that the observer is inevitably and inexorably a part of what he observes, so that what the researcher confronts is 'reality' as apprehended through his own particular prism of perception, and what he gathers as results are artefacts of the process of his observation (see Wiener 1949, p. 191). The research process is an interactive one, and the researcher, the observer, is at one and the same time an interactant, a part of the field of events under observation. Any interpretation of the information accrued, therefore, must somehow come to terms with the fact that far from being 'things-in-themselves', true for all places and all times, data are epiphenomena of their means of acquisition and their framework of representation. If there is no 'immaculate perception', and there are 'no facts, only interpretations', as adumbrated by Nietzsche (1911) on the cusp of the twentieth century, then research observations, interpretations and generalisations are not so readily distinguishable from beliefs, hypotheses and evaluations (see John MacDonald, this volume).

If there is a growing recognition in the natural sciences that 'proofs' are learnt and respected practices common to a paradigm, and 'truth' to a significant degree 'a matter of fit: fit to what is referred to in one way or another, or to other renderings, or to modes and manners of organisation' (Goodman 1978, p. 138), then anthropology has also come to accept that 'ethnographic reality is actively constructed, not to say invented' (Dumont 1978, p. 66). To write an authentic anthropological text is less to represent an absolute reality than to fabricate a fit of a particular generic kind between two types of conventional activity (exchanging spoken words and arranging written words), and hence to 'write' social reality. The 'truth' of anthropological accounts, in a celebrated formulation by Roy Wagner, is that anthropologists invent a culture for their informants: here is 'what they imagine to be a plausible explanation of what they understand them generally to have been doing' (1977, pp. 500–501).

This conclusion remains controversial, nonetheless, and much anthropological debate continues to occur concerning the nature of research processes, of research results, and of the presenting and appreciating of information. What should anthropology represent itself as if not a 'generalising science' (see Ingold 1997)? Surely it is more than merely 'a collection of travellers' tales' (Louch 1966, p. 160)? For some, however, this ambiguity and uncertainty is all grist to the anthropological mill. Anthropology – 'the most humanistic of the social sciences, the most scientific of the humanities' – has never been comfortably placed within certain categories of disciplinary knowledge, and, indeed, has seen its project as the exploration, and the calling into question, of conventional and disciplinary divisions as such. Anthropology was 'born omniform', Clifford Geertz asserts (1983, p. 21), and should refuse to be bound or restricted by the preconceptions of categorial knowledge. In seeking as complex an appreciation of experience as possible, an appreciation of the ambiguities concerning the nature of knowledge and truth should make anthropology 'more like itself' (see Rapport 1997a).

This certainly became Sir Edmund Leach's message. Drawing inspiration from the eighteenth-century philosopher–scientist Giambattista Vico, Leach set great store by the facility of an anthropologist's 'artistic imagination' (1982, p. 53). For Vico, the human imagination was to be regarded as a primary tool in a 'new science', which sought to understand the real as opposed to the outwardly observable nature of a human engagement with its environment. Such real knowledge called for an attempted entering into the minds of other people; so that one came to know not only *that* (Caesar was dead) or *how* (to ride a bike) but *what it was like* (to be poor, to be in love, to belong to a community). Moreover, it was in the nature of this imaginative knowing, or *fantasia*, that it was not analysable except in terms of itself, and it could not be identified except by examples.

Furthermore, for Leach, since 'the only ego I know at first hand is my own' (1989, p. 138), anthropological research was to be conceived of as a subjective process whose 'data' represented 'a kind of harmonic projection of the observer's own personality' (1984, p. 22). Inevitably, each anthropologist saw something which no other would recognise. But this still made the results of anthropological research admissible as knowledge because the aim was not 'objective truth' but 'insight' into behaviour, one's own as well as others': a 'quality of deep understanding' equivalent to 'fully understanding the nuances of a language [as opposed to] simply knowing the dictionary glosses of individual words' (1982, p. 52). This made anthropological writings 'interesting in themselves' – full of meaning, intended and unintended – and not revelatory of 'the external world' so much as of the author's reactions and interactions with it (1984, p. 22).

In this Leach comes close to the tenor of suggestions by physics Nobel-laureate Ilya Prigogine (1989). For Prigogine, an appreciation of the instability and creativity inherent in our world, the impossibility of absolute control or precise forecasting, and a clearer view of the place of human activity-within-the-world, now bring the projects of natural science and social science close to one another. In both, old notions of determinism, materialism and reductionism, of knowledge as omniscient and timeless, must give way to 'a narrative element' in the way we conceive of our knowledge, represent it, and act upon its implications. For, '[i]n effect, all human and social interaction and all literature is the expression of uncertainty about the future, and of a construction of the future' (1989, p. 389).

An emphasis on narrative in turn spurs a treating of culture and society and their representation as 'personal documents'. As a generic category of writing which includes diaries, autobiographies, life histories and letters (Allport 1942), personal documents have long had a respected place in certain, more humanistic versions of anthropological practice. What is different now, perhaps, is a matter of emphasis and evaluation. There is an appreciation of the 'personal document' of society and culture not as a partial component, as a biased version, as an over-determined manifestation, as false consciousness, or whatever, but as all there is. In a fitting reversal, it is recognised that only by way of the personal documentation of individual naming do society and culture take their place in history (cf. Atkinson 1993, p. 7).

It is to the personal document of a porter's life amid the hierarchical institution of a modern state hospital that this chapter now turns.

METHOD: PERSONAL DOCUMENT VIA PARTICIPANT-OBSERVATION

Bob carries himself distinctively as he bestrides the corridors, offices and wards of Hospital X. His porter's uniform of blue fabric trousers and yellow polo-shirt (with name tag on the left breast) are tightly stretched across a bodybuilder's frame, in particular chest and neck. Bob has well-developed trapezius and latissimus dorsi muscles, as well as pectorals and deltoids. And he holds them with a certain tightness and expansiveness through the day. With his blond hair in crew-cut style, his glasses magnifying a slight squint in his eye, and a slight stoop in his posture, Bob – 'Bob, SUPPORT SERVICES' – is a readily identifiable figure at Hospital X.

Hospital X is a major teaching hospital, furnished with a wide range of medical specialisms, in a large town in the east of Scotland. State-funded, it caters to an increasingly large catchment area, dealing with all manner of medical need from physical to psychological, surgery to therapy, accident-and-emergency to long-term care. Hospital X has thousands of employees, among whom are more than 130 porters. Porters are not medically trained; hence, in a setting geared to the privileging of medical know-how and skill, the ministering and the administration of medical expertise, porters occupy a lowly position. 'You might think porters are a small cog in a large machine', I was told by a portering sub-manager during my induction-morning to the job, 'but don't think you're nothing just because people say you are. People might say you're "just a porter" but it's not true; no part of the hospital could run without you (the same with domestics)'.[2] In practice, much exchange is orchestrated hierarchically, with porters and domestics engaged in routine practices regarded as less precious than those of clerks, carpenters, laboratory technicians, nurses, doctors (students, surgeons and consultants) and administrators. Porters are involved in tasks calling for physical stamina, even strength, more than any other criteria. They ferry patients (and sometimes visitors) across the hospital, in wheelchairs, beds and trolleys; they deliver mail within the hospital; they carry body parts and samples of bodily substances between different parts of the hospital complex; they transport dead bodies from hospital ward to mortuary; and they act as security personnel, policing the boundaries between hospital and outside world. (Interestingly, the English word 'porter' has a dual etymology deriving from the Latin word *portiarius*, a door-keeper, gate-keeper or janitor, and also from the Latin *portare*, to carry.)

By focusing on Bob as an individual case study, I would explore the ways in which this institutional structure is animated and lived – comes alive – in the context of a particular person's life. Bob might be employed as a porter at Hospital X but he is also a bodybuilder. And it is as a bodybuilder, I shall argue, that he fills out his porter's uniform and occupies the plant, fulfilling his portering duties. In elucidating how Bob speaks and acts and reflects upon his time in the hospital as well as outside it, I would reflect upon the ways and extent to which the nature of the hospital as a social institution deploying categories of social distinction and hierarchy can be said to be obviated by Bob's acts of will. Certainly, I would hope to show how the boundaries between the hospital and the outside world, as between the work environment and the time and space of recreation and 'leisure' beyond it, are routinely permeated by Bob's actions and intentions. What, in contrast, might be said to retain an integrity is Bob's body, as a project of his personal development, means and manifestation of his being and becoming (see Rapport 2003).

The wider implications of the case study concern a refocusing of social-scientific attention: less on bodies-in-institutions than on bodies-in-between. Stretching the metaphor, here is the body *per se* as porter: carrying the energy and agency by which institutions are animated, gate-keeper to the meanings and identities they come to host.

RESULTS: BOB, HOSPITAL BODYBUILDER

I first met Bob during the two-week period of 'shadowing' another, more experienced porter – accompanying him on his round of tasks – which followed my morning of induction into the job. Bob and I had taken a trolley down to a ward to collect a patient for an ambulance trip to another institution and were now waiting while the nurses (behind closed curtains) transferred the patient to the trolley from his bed. 'Don't work too hard at this job,' Bob began. 'The others in the buckie [the porters' lodge] don't so why should you? And when you've done a job, go for a walk; don't go back to front door straight away . . . But it's not a bad job, like, not too hard'. A domestic cleaner, languidly pushing a broom, hears Bob's talk and wanders over to us: 'New porter?' she says to Bob, and half to me. I smile and nod. 'How many have they taken on?' 'Six,' Bob explains, 'but one has already gone to Hospital Y [another hospital in the area], and few of the others will stay; three, maybe, there's always a fast turnover.' 'Will you stay?' the domestic asks me directly. 'Probably,' I mumble, smile, and look away. She's been here 16 years, the domestic explains to both of us, and she still gets lost in the laboratory block sometimes; all the corridors look the same! 'That's shite,' says Bob to her in reply. 'It's really not so hard to get round, Nigel. Don't listen to her. And you don't get lost, it's just talk: she never really got lost. How long did you say you'd been here!?' Bob grins and the domestic does too, while still insisting that she does lose herself by the 'labs'.

Collecting our patient, Bob and I leave the ward. 'The lab block is really not hard,' Bob continues. 'I've been working here about a year, though only a few months of that as a front-door porter; so I don't know my way around as well as I could, but it's still only occasionally that you get lost.' I ask him what he did before he was on the front door. 'I used to be on security, at the reception desk. If there was violence, or an incident where someone got unruly, they'd call me. But it was a good number, and not much happened. A few incidents: visitors or patients getting violent. Just 'cos of drink usually . . . Now never take a patient onto Pipe Street,' Bob changes tack as we pass the entrance to that part of the hospital where the extensive heating and ventilation pipe systems run, 'That's an instant sacking!' I tell Bob I have heard about Pipe Street from Pat, the portering manager who ran my induction course: he said I was to report it immediately if ever I saw vermin there. 'Vermin!' Bob is aghast, 'In Pipe Street?! Huh! Pat is full of shite.'

I have taken time over this first exchange with Bob because it introduces nicely a number of themes that Bob would dwell on in our later interactions, as well as the forthright manner of his delivery. Bob would maintain his own point of view; also he would distance himself from the workaday banter of the hospital employees, which could not be taken at face value as the truth; he would get away with not working hard if he could; and he would disparage both the portering management and the rest of the porters as was necessary to maintain his own interests and his distance from them.

For instance, it was not long after the above conversation that Bob confided in me that while most were okay, there were 'some c**** here among the porters' – as anywhere, he supposed. In part this was for my benefit; if I, a professor of anthropology, was deigning to spend some time among a less reliable and a less sophisticated set, then, he wanted me to know, he was too, in a way. Hence, in seeing me perusing the tabloid newspapers which were the porters' daily fare, in their rest room, Bob advised me: 'Don't read that, Nigel. The *Sun* and [*The Daily*] *Record* are all crap.' These seem to me complex utterances. In part Bob wanted to assure me that he recognised the gulf between my usual social milieu and this, and that he too partook of something of the former (he had his education and his middle-class associates); he also wanted me to remain unsullied, perhaps, as a reminder to him – a tangible link – of his more proper existence elsewhere. But this was also part of Bob's routine speaking *persona* when engaging with porters at large. Almost in a challenging way, and even when surrounded by a roomful, Bob would distinguish himself:

NIGEL: Are you coming on the porters' night out, Bob?
BOB: No. It's not my thing. I don't like quite a number of them even when they're sober! Drunk and I'd probably want to strangle them!

And Bob would be disparaging:

> Porters are all a bunch of f****** drunks. That's the main qualification for the job! 'How much do you drink?' 'As much as my belly will take! More again, after I'm sick!' [he laughs] You could write a book about this lot, Nigel; it would sell millions. The things you could say! I could feed you the information . . . They're drunken, sexist, dirty, skiving . . .

I think Bob enjoyed the uncertainty his fellows must have felt regarding how much of an insider Bob saw himself as being, or wanted to be. My feeling though is that the routine stance he set himself was on the edge, such as when he impugned the physicality of the porter's trade and denied the need for it to be, in Hospital X, almost exclusively male:

> But the porters are so sexist [i e. exclusively male sex]. And I don't know why. There is nothing porters do that women could not. In fact, no job that men do is impossible for women to do – or only those few using extreme strength.

If anyone was to think portering was hard physical graft, I understand Bob to be implying, they should consider the extremities that bodybuilding treats.

Bob summed up for me his feelings towards the rest of the porters one day like this:

> I don't like many of the porters in the hospital, Nigel. After work I don't want to see them. I mean, if I saw them downtown and they were in trouble, of course I'd help: I'd wade in, no question. 'Cos they're my work-mates. But they also drive me mad. They are so limited. And their conversation is so boring. Haven't you noticed? It's a three-way conversation with them: betting, drinking, shagging women. That's all they talk about, all the time. And, you know, if you came back in five years you'd find the same people having *exactly* the same conversations!

Not that Bob's distancing himself from the portering staff entailed seeing himself as any closer to, or openly sympathetic of, the management, it should be made clear. 'Managerial scum' was his comment on discovering that the dates he requested for his annual leave had not been granted. It was a regular refrain that management were 'messing him about', and that the way they allocated him jobs and shifts 'was not right'.

One day I found Bob in the porters' lodge in a distracted mood, wearing civilian clothes; inspecting next week's schedule, he had found that he had been given yet more nights. 'Where is Fred [the shop steward]?' he demands of the portering charge-hand, 'And who's his replacement shop steward if he's away?' Bob finally agrees with the charge-hand that he should go 'upstairs' now and talk to Davy, the relevant sub-manager, about it personally. Some days later he tells me what happened: how he 'got aggressive' when he went to complain about his shifts, actually seeing Sue, the manager, and how she later complained to Davy [the sub-manager] that she had felt scared when faced by him; physically intimidated. 'And since that day,' Bob concluded with a satisfied grin, 'they've both given me a wide berth. I may work here but they leave me alone! They both learnt that they can't just take me for granted!'

What gave Bob this otherness to his hospital *persona* – the reason neither management nor porters could 'take him for granted' – I would argue, was that his sense of self, and a confident public identity which Bob intended in many ways to be larger than life, derived from his practice as a bodybuilder. Distant from the porters and their world, it was his body, its changing capacities and proclivities, to which he was close.

Conversation between him and me soon routinely turned to bodybuilding; it was visibly apparent the time and energy that Bob devoted to the practice, as I say, while, at least between the ages of 14 and 29, it had also been a major preoccupation of mine. Bob first introduced his bodybuilding to me in this way:

BOB: I'm an oddity, Nigel. Most porters have no hobbies outside work; they just work and booze. But I don't drink. I used to, but not any more, not for 8 years or so . . . And I'm just back to working my legs. 'Cos I injured them 2 years ago; I had my cartilage scraped – there's none there now – and my bones were getting stuck in one position. I couldn't bend my knee. So I had an operation. In fact, I had my first work-out last night! Yeah! And now it feels strange, bouncy, when I walk.

NIGEL: You better take it easy at first, you know.

BOB: I'm certainly gonna begin slowly; I'd never be one to rush things you know, and risk more injury. It's just crazy doing that . . . So I just began with some leg-raise machine . . . But you know my weight has gone down to 14,4!

NIGEL: What was it?

BOB: 15,2. So I wanna start putting it on again . . . I do a 9-week protein blitz, then rest the body for 3 weeks and get the system back to normal. I'm about to start a blitz again now.

NIGEL: What d'you take?

BOB: Vitamin and protein supplements. Centrum [I look blank]. Not heard of it? I'm surprised. It's like HMB. Heard of that? [I nod weakly.] But it's cheaper 'cos it's not so effective.

NIGEL: What does it cost?

BOB: 18 quid, and that lasts me about a month . . . But you gotta take supplements if you wanna get bigger; eating will not do it by itself. And I eat an enormous amount too and do all my own cooking. [I look quizzical.] Oh, yes; I can't trust anyone else to do it. Or expect them to!

NIGEL: How about steroids?

BOB: No. I wouldn't know where to get them. And I'd be worried about side effects. Like, they say they can make you go deaf.

What becomes clear, however, as Bob and I talk more regularly is that the above represents what might be called the strong or confident or proud position – the strong thesis – of Bob's bodybuilding habit, and that actually its terms are the subject of a struggle in his life. What will it take to maintain himself at the extreme? His training, his diet, his weight, his loosenings or lapses of control over these facets of his bodily regimen, are frequently aired.

There is, for instance, the question of sleep, also of being in bed as against being in the gym training. On the one hand, Bob insists he can cope with two or three hours' sleep and does not mind early shifts at the hospital or having only a few hours of sleep between shifts; and this can go on for a number of days before he starts noticing a lack of ability to concentrate. Recently, he recalls, he finished a weekend shift and went straight on to a party and felt fine, even though it meant some 72 hours without proper sleep. When he goes training, meanwhile, 'he really trains'; usually it means a session from 5 p.m. until 10.30 p.m. On the other hand, Bob muses how he loves his bed and is just too lazy. He can go to bed at about midnight after an evening shift and then sleep for 16 hours – waking up around 8 a.m., having a sandwich and a drink, and then going back to bed to sleep. This can mean that he misses the work-outs that he intended for himself; it also entails Bob elaborating on what happens when he misses sleep: his 'inability to concentrate' means that he feels physically exhausted and shaky, and 'his head shuts down'.

The same is true as regards diet. He wants to put on weight and knows how important intake of the right foods is towards this end; he had today, for instance, three carefully prepared breakfasts (the best meal): a drink of raw eggs, then Weetabix, and then cooked eggs. After this morning's meal he went out and did a new circuit, training new muscle groups, before his afternoon hospital shift, and it felt very good; tomorrow morning when he wakes up he will feel really stiff, properly sore. 'Everything is a mental attitude,' Bob explains, putting his hands up besides his eyes (like blinkers) and taking them forwards as if tracing a straight course ahead: 'losing, gaining weight, all of it; if you train without the right attitude you just get injured.' But then, accepting chocolate from another porter in the buckie, after a brief struggle with his conscience, Bob also admits that he's weak: and while other people might not be able to see him putting on weight where it should not be, on his belly and his sides, he can. Moreover, his knee has recently given out again which means no more weight-training for a while; his weight has dipped further, to 14 stones 2 pounds.

In the course of Bob's struggles with himself it seems at times that he sees through the discourse or mantra of bodybuilding to a real body of his, under-neath, which has its own rhythms:

> I like being 14,2, Nigel. I was taking in too much protein, and the body can only absorb so much. After that it becomes fat. You know my body-fat percentage was 30% [he grins and shakes his head incredulously]! I was carrying it all in my back.

And again, while insisting that he would 'never dream' of taking drugs – 'does not do steroids', 'would never put a needle into himself', 'would NEVER mess with needles' – Bob also recognises that everything is a steroid of some sort, all these supplements which bodybuilders use are: 'even Centrum!'.

Fixing his focus on his body, its tendencies and his work on it, Bob removes himself cognitively and socially from encompassment by the institution of the hospital, its personnel and relationships. But what this leads him into, it now appears, is a struggle which Bob does not always win, nor one he seems always to want to. There are moments when he appears pleased about the laziness he can accord the rest of the porters, their hobby-less state, for the resort, the fall-back position it affords him – eager, for instance, for chocolate. At other times Bob's body seems to represent a middle way and an integrity which distin-guishes him from all institutional discourse: that of the bodybuilders and their gym as well as the porters and the hospital. For it is also the case that body-building involves Bob in other sets of relations with which he can seem equally ambivalent:

> I was told last year that I had great Middle Deltoids and that they could be cham-pionship material, but since then my weights and my motivation have gone right down! Isn't that weird? You'd think it would be the opposite . . . But I've been in here [at the gym] four times in the past two months. I just can't motivate myself, Nigel. But I know that if I don't train properly, eat properly, take supplements, and the rest, I'll not grow and the whole thing won't be worth doing.

This exchange took place while Bob and I were working-out at his regular gym; it is perhaps time to bring Bob's relations outside the hospital into some-what clearer focus.

He is very independent, Bob tells me, and has lived in his own house since he was 16. Now he is 33, and it's a complicated arrangement but – 'until she kicks him out!' – he lives with his girlfriend and looks after not his own two kids (whom he has hardly seen for six years) but her kids' kids; she has a girl and a boy and they each have a boy. She's a bit older than him – mid-forties – and works as a child counsellor. In fact, he and his girlfriend are really like chalk and cheese. Take diet, for instance: he eats more in a day than she does in a week – literally. She can get by on a packet of crisps, a day; seven in a week! She eats nothing at all. If she's eating her occasional steak or chicken he'll eat with her but otherwise, even if she's just eating eggs or some such rubbish (since you can't put on weight just with eggs), he'll eat separately.

Watching Bob and his girlfriend, Moira, together it is clear that their difference in eating habits is a regular part of their joint discourse. When Bob talks about Moira's diet, moreover, it is not with distaste; more amazement, even pride. Because, she doesn't starve herself, he assures me, and she isn't dieting, and she has a great body – not too thin; it's just that she has never needed to eat, since she was small. Occasionally, these days, she feels a bit funny – the ageing process – and then he advises her that she must take vitamin supplements too, like him.

On the other hand, Moira is not too keen on him putting on a lot more muscle either; she says it's like cuddling a rock. She says the paraphernalia of bodybuilding competitions – the suntan lotion and the rest; pectoral muscles being tensed – makes her feel like vomiting. Bob thinks, however, that she'll come around. After all, he employs a personal trainer – you have to if you are a serious lifter – and would like to compete at National Juniors level, even though what he's most into is shape: bodybuilding as distinct from weightlifting.

When I first met Bob he worked out at a gym called 'Healthy Bodies', he told me. There were some very big guys there but he had the nicest shape. But there were also coming to be too many distractions there – women in leotards – so he decided to change gyms. After all, he never found it hard to settle into a new place or make friends, and 'The Leisure Centre' was no 'fitness club' with posers and what have you, but only for those seriously into weights. He was one of the smallest and one of the weakest guys who now trained there, some of whom (whose photographs adorned the walls) had won bodybuilding championships. Of the ten lads he trained with he was certainly in the lower five. The best, indeed, was a young lad – only small, 11 stone or so at first, then moved up to 13 – who could be a champ. He lifted championship weights – benching 140 kilos, squatting 130 – and might break the Scottish record one day, even the British one.

Some months after Bob first told me about his young friend, the possible champ, I heard about him again. But now Bob added that after moving up from 11 stone to 13:

he then went up to 15 stone. And he said he was one big scab, just full of pus. And that if you pressed him he would explode: all the pus would escape. Now I've not seen him for an age . . . He might be dead! Aye, he'll be dead.

What I take this to signify is Bob displaying the same kind of internal struggle concerning the relationships that surround his bodybuilding as we found in the case of his bodily regimen, as well as in the case of the porters. His girlfriend – chalk to his cheese – might well throw him out; he is smaller and weaker than most he trains with, but does he want to become like them anyway if winning championships entails endangering the body with drugs, risking injury, infection, life itself? He is told he is championship material but body shape is what he most works for – although this is something, too, that his girlfriend claims not to appreciate.

In other words, relationships to do with his bodybuilding, and concerning people beyond the hospital – girlfriend, personal trainer, training buddies – who might seem to provide an alternative to hospital institutionalism and its personnel, appear, on closer inspection, to be no more central to Bob's life; or rather they provide no more fixed a focal point. What perhaps they do afford is a counterweight, a place for Bob to go for social and emotional support, but not a place in which Bob needs to stay. In the same way, then, that Bob points up the contradictions in the dietary regimen of bodybuilding to which he episodically submits himself – everything is really a drug, a steroid, even Centrum – he also sees through the relationships in which bodybuilding involves him and points out their shortcomings.

Let me finish an ethnographic account of Bob's bodybuilding, then, by coming full circle and returning to two incidents in the milieu of the hospital. Having decried most of his porter colleagues for having no hobbies outside work beyond boozing, it was interesting to see Bob return a compliment one day; after being greeted by one of the charge-hands by the welcome shout of 'Here's Steroids!', Bob retorted that the charge-hand's nickname was 'Mighty Mouse' because he too worked out – in fact, Bob joked with me, it was the charge-hand who got him his steroids in the first place! And again, having laughingly and repeatedly insisted to a nurse that he knew that her son planned to get married – however well she might claim to know her son and his plans and deny Bob's charge – Bob explained to me he was just 'winding her up' because her son was someone he loved to tease. Her son worked at the Reception at Bob's gym – a big lad himself – and Bob could not wait to hear how she went home and he was forced to deny it: ' "That bastard, Bob", he'll go!' In short, what Bob most liked to be, I would conclude, was not a bodybuilder as such, far less a hospital porter, but a bodybuilder in the hospital: 'Bob, Hospital Bodybuilder'.

ANALYSIS: THE IMPORTANCE OF 'ELSEWHERE'

I was in my early thirties when I began to find bodybuilding tedious; establishing myself in new gyms as I moved between towns and jobs, keeping up the same levels of accomplishment – never mind improvement – felt increasingly more like work than recreation. Bob professed not to mind moving between gyms and groups of lifters and re-establishing himself, but at 33 he too seemed to be finding the required effort and motivation harder to come by. Evidently, looking at his body, he had put in the time in the past, and he was still massively muscled; when we worked out together in his gym our circuits were too different – in particular exercises (in muscle groups exercised) and in weights lifted – for me really to serve as his partner and 'spotter'. However, what I have argued is that not only did Bob use bodybuilding as means to distance himself, cognitively and socially, from the hospital and the rest of the porters but also that Bob was pleased, on occasion, to know himself as 'Steroids' *in* the hospital: as the hospital's bodybuilder, even though at the same time he knew that he slept rather than worked-out, ate chocolate and put down fat deposits on his back. Bob's bodybuilding seemed intimately connected with a multiplying of identities and milieux, and a juggling and translocation among them.

In his poem, 'The Importance of Elsewhere', Philip Larkin describes his alienation from the milieux in England in which he lives (1990, p. 104; also see Rapport 2000). It is not that he finds himself a stranger, as he does, say, in Ireland. In fact, quite the opposite; he is able to accommodate himself to visiting Ireland *because* there he is 'separate' and things should feel strange: 'since it was not home, /Strangeness made sense'. But living in England he has no such excuse for his loneliness and alone-ness; these are meant to be his 'customs and establishments'. 'Here', Larkin concludes, 'no elsewhere underwrites my existence'.

Erving Goffman has written famously and (by and large) convincingly about the characteristics of what he termed 'total institutions': social environments, from prisons to boarding schools to hospitals, where a number of individuals 'together lead an enclosed, formally administered round of life' (1961, p. 11). On arrival in the institution, individuals find their senses of self 'mortified': 'the boundary that the individual places between his being and the environment is invaded and the embodiment of self profaned' (1961, p. 32). Their conceptions of self no longer supported by everyday social arrangements, individuals-in-the-institution embark upon new and radically altered, alienating, moral careers: ones of curtailment and dispossession, disfigurement and violation. Encompassed by the institution – their time and interests captured by the institutional regimen provided them – they find every aspect of their lives overwritten. More recently, Michel Foucault (1977) has generalised upon these insights and seen bodies 'totally imprinted by history' everywhere. Not only the inmates (the prisoners, school-children and patients) but also the employees of total institutions (the warders, teachers and medics) find themselves mortified and alienated. And more than this, since, according to Foucault, identity and sense of self are themselves the product of discourse, there is never a time when 'the laws of individual desire, the forms of individual language, the rules of individual actions, and the play of individual mythical and imaginative discourses' are not overwritten and over-determined in this way (1972, p. 22).

The indiscriminateness of Foucault's notions, whereby the 'governmentality' (1977) of discourse is responsible for all identity, individual or other, seemingly free or constrained, supposedly gratifying or alienating, is a far cry from Goffman's more humanistic vision wherein institutions are something one can imagine individuals entering and leaving. Nevertheless, the way Foucault connects up life in a so-called institution to that in the milieux beyond it is useful for this discussion. For my own argument would be that what we see Bob effecting through his bodybuilding is a measure of control over his identity and a maintaining of a sense of integrity concerning his bodily self whether in the hospital or out, or in negotiating the transition between. As 'hospital bodybuilder' Bob compassed or contained a sense of elsewhere within himself, and as such was never contained, alienated or overwritten by the locale in which he found himself – hospital, gym or wherever. He moved between the work of the hospital and the 'leisure' of the gym, between the 'work' of the gym and the 'leisure' of the hospital, and between the work of a bodily regimen and the leisure of luxuriating his body in chocolate and sleep. He could be said to be at home in keeping on the move between institutional or discursive fixities (see Rapport & Dawson 1998). '[N]either here nor there', Bob's home was *both* here *and* there – an amalgam, a pastiche, a performance' (Bammer 1992, p. ix). What I want to reiterate, however, is that this amalgam, pastiche and transitive performance which Bob practised – which, indeed, Bob *embodied* since it was his body that was the focus of so much of his attention in the construction of his identity – was his project not his alienation. Bob eluded the control of the institution, from the singularity of discourse and setting as such, with a bodily focus by which he came to contain multitudes ('elsewheres') within himself: weightlifter, porter, luxurist.

Finally, and despite his protestations to the contrary, Bob's having a hobby, a leisure pursuit that afforded him cognitive distance from workmates and place of work, was not something peculiar or special to him. Among the porters of Hospital X it may even have been something of a norm (Rapport 2002). A number of younger porters were involved in rock bands; others sold cut-price videos, CDs and tapes, cigarettes and whisky; for a great many, watching and playing football was the most important thing in the week; for others it was the time spent drinking in the local pubs and clubs, the local watering-hole, 'The Hilltop', being only 100 metres from the hospital door. For other porters again, I would say, time in the hospital was passed by it being itself turned into a pursuit of 'leisure': of practical jokes, of bantering or 'good crack', of smoking and eating, of wasting time.

We have heard how, for Bob, there was a slippage, a flexibility, regarding the status of hospital and gym as either 'work' or 'leisure'. Albeit that the hospital was where he got paid – and to assure himself of his wages he could not decide to sleep through his shift-time as he could his time for work-outs – his attitude to the hospital as it related to the gym was variable. He both escaped from the hospital as work place to the recreational space of the gym, and he escaped from the rigours of the gym to the relaxation of the hospital; he also escaped from working on his body to luxuriating in it. In conclusion, I would say, this too was not Bob's special preserve. 'Work' and 'leisure' among the porters of Hospital X pertained not to certain fixed times or locations nor to certain circumscribed practices; rather, they were attitudes, frames of mind, by which times, locations and practices were approached. Other porters might not be serious bodybuilders like Bob, but in their singing, their drinking, their foot-balling, their entrepreneurialism and their sedition – their 'disciplined' prac-tising of these – they provided themselves with elsewheres whereby their lives and their bodies were imprinted by their intentions, and where 'work' and 'leisure' significantly pertained to their own constructions of routine and recre-ation, and their own jugglings of identity.

DISCUSSION: TOWARDS A 'PERFECT' BIOGRAPHY

From qualitative versus quantitative methods of knowledge acquisition, this chapter moved to issues of foregrounding the narrative nature of a human being-in-the-world, and coming to terms with knowledge-processes that were constructive and interpretational. The growth of such self-consciousness in anthropology – as both epistemology and representation – has changed radic-ally the nature of the disciplinary endeavour: given it a 'literary turn' (Rapport 1994). As urged by Rodney Needham (1978, pp. 75–76): a 'counsel of perfection' might now see anthropologists reassessing their tasks, their standards and their ambitions, and contemplating what the discipline might become if it were to break free from its present academicism. Might not anthropology one day achieve something possessing the humane significance of metaphysics and art, Needham ponders, if ethnographic interpretations were written with the imaginative acuity, the empathetic penetration, and the literary artistry of a George Eliot, a Dostoyevsky or a Virginia Woolf?

Anthropological opinion remains divided, however, concerning what might be described as the collapse of objectivity as a tenet in natural science (à la Heisenberg and Prigogine) and its implications for the discipline. Some see the collapse as a challenge, others as a temporary aberration to be lamented and overcome. Sharing Needham's vision, for instance, are Watson and Watson-Franke (1985, pp. 96–97, 133), for whom:

> [m]uch ethnographic research lacks a true feeling for human life as it is subjec-tively experienced by individuals. We know the richness and complexity of our own inner life, and when we compare this to the many tedious, dehumanizing accounts of life in other cultures . . . we may feel an acute sense of disinterest and even outright alienation. . . . All too often the real things seem to get lost in the obfuscation of the investigator playing God with his constructs. . . . To understand the individual in his human fullness we must therefore suspend total commitment to our scientific preconceptions and enter into a dialogue with the life history.

Watson and Watson-Franke would urge a greater appreciation in anthropology of the narrative and life-history, the personal document, as a means to restore to the individual actor (anthropological researcher and subject) a measure of his lost integrity, dignity and significance. For such personal documentation may be understood both as an act by which the individual constitutes his social-experiential environment, and one by which the anthropologist is able to access the individual in the act of managing his self-defined transactions with reality. While, they suggest, social science has tended to come to grips with experience by robbing it of its unique richness and fluidity, privileging models, quantities and the experimental testing of hypotheses, and translating experience into static and essential abstractions ('culture', 'social structure', *'habitus'* etc.), a narrative of personal documents gives onto that subjective consciousness through which the individual articulates his world. In sum, through a personal documentation the anthropologist can do justice to 'the flow of subjective experience', others' and his own, to a phenomenal consciousness as the individual himself experiences it (Watson & Watson-Franke 1985, p. 97).

For others, such as James Weiner (1995), the value of personal narratives in anthropology remains low and their use is to be disparaged, for a focus on personal documents prescribes an unnecessarily narrow understanding of culture, and a reduction of social life to text. Whereas society and culture are significantly more than the stories individuals tell of them: to wit, there is the contrast between what is told and what is done, between 'what language avers and what behaviour reveals' (Weiner 1995, p. 5). Moreover, social practices and cultural knowledges are unevenly and restrictedly distributed, and an isolating of any one person's account will thus represent a partial understanding of the total socio-cultural repertoire of what is known. At best, Weiner concludes, 'narrated memoirs' serve to distinguish the rather feeble methodology of the oral historian from that of the social scientist; unlike the oral historian (but more like the psychoanalyst), the anthropologist should socially situate the individual narrator so as to reveal influences and constraints upon his personal documentation (whether in speech or in action) of which he himself may be unaware.

One might question, however, whether Weiner's view of the objectivity of science and culture, and the anthropology that might emanate from their study, is outmoded. Certainly, it is arguable that it is not 'a culture' that possesses a total repertoire of things known, in the way that Weiner would portray, but rather individuals who create and possess an ongoing multitude of diverse and discrepant knowledges that they put to use in the animation of sociocultural forms. And while it is true that there is more to observe than 'stories about social life', it is not true that these other things (from theories to sensations) are any less personal or any more objectively accessible. They are also personal documents, no less interpreted and hence narrated by the individual, and no more properly or hegemonically determinable by another. What lies beyond an individual's narrations, in short, are other narrations – by the same individual and by others. The anthropologist can collect and juxtapose these in his description-analysis – as may the oral historian – but one narrative does not necessarily 'situate' another, does not give onto a superior awareness.

Because of the novelist's command of the personal life of the individual, and the former's desire to connect the externally observable with the internally responsible, E. M. Forster (1984) opined that literature was 'truer' than social science. For, while each person knew from experience that there was much beyond the 'outer' evidence of observation, and while the social scientist claimed to be equally concerned to record human character, the latter appeared content to restrict himself to what could be known of its existence from scouring 'the exterior surface' of social life only, and to what could approximately be deduced from people's actions, words and gestures. Only the novelist appeared determined to accrue a fuller knowledge, and seek out 'the hidden life at its [individual] source' (Forster 1984, pp. 55–56).

Increasingly, the distinction Forster would make no longer stands. Anthropologists admit that novelists have dealt better than social scientists in the past with 'the subtleties, inflections and varieties of individual consciousness which are concealed by the categorical masks' of membership in social and cultural groups (Cohen 1994, p. 180), and there are attempts in growing numbers to remedy the practice. In an anthropology *of* personal documentation, and an anthropology *as* personal documentation, the impersonalising impulses of an earlier social science are eschewed (Rapport 1997b). In 'ethnographies of the particular' (Abu-Lughod 1991, p. 138), the complexity of individual experience its elusiveness to the researcher and to the individual alike (cf. Atkinson 2000) – is no longer necessarily reduced, abstracted, typified or overwritten.

ACKNOWLEDGEMENTS

The research on which this chapter reports was funded by the Leverhulme Trust (grant no. XCHL48), under the aegis of their 'Nations and Regions' programme, and part of the 'Constitutional Change and Identity' project convened by Professor David McCrone of Edinburgh University.

I am grateful to Professor John Atkinson for convivial engagements across divides of distance and discipline as the research was conducted.

NOTES

1. 'Social anthropology' was the name of the discipline that developed in Britain during the twentieth century and 'cultural anthropology' that in North America. Due to the growth of centres of anthropological practice (continental Europe, Australasia, Israel, India) and the increasing overlap in their enterprises – encompassing both

an appreciation of social structure and the institutional, and the provenance of the symbological – the convention has grown to refer, as I do here, to 'sociocultural anthropology'.
2. Participant-observation was conducted 'in role'. With the permission of the hospital authorities, the portering charge-hands and union, I undertook, in a voluntary capacity, the day-to-day shift work of a porter over a period of nine months (followed by three months of broader interviewing). I hoped as far as possible to insinuate myself into a porter's life-world at Hospital X (and, to a lesser extent, outside the hospital too) by doing as and what other porters did. My fieldwork practice was not to tape-record informants but yet to aim for a detailed accounting of interactions I witnessed. As soon as possible after an interaction's end I would discreetly transcribe key words onto paper, for a full writing-up in my journal later.

REFERENCES

Abu-Lughod, L. (1991) Writing against culture. In R. Fox (ed.) *Recapturing Anthropology*. School of American Research Press, Sante Fe, NM.
Allport, G. (1942) *The Use of Personal Documents in Psychological Science*. Social Science Research Council, New York.
Atkinson, J. (1993) When somebody knows my name. *Radix* October, p. 7.
Atkinson, J. (2000) *Nursing Homeless Men: A Study of Proactive Intervention*. John Wiley & Sons, Chichester.
Bammer, A. (1992) Editorial. *New Formations* special edition: The Question of 'Home' **2**(2): 1–24.
Cohen, A. P. (1994) *Self Consciousness. An Alternative Anthropology of Identity*. Routledge, London.
Dumont, J.-P. (1978) *The Headman and I*. University of Texas Press, Austin, TX.
Forster, E. M. (1984) *Aspects of the Novel*. Penguin, Harmondsworth.
Foucault, M. (1972) *The Archaeology of Knowledge*. Harper, New York.
Foucault, M. (1977) *Discipline and Punish*. Pantheon, New York.
Geertz, C. (1983) *Local Knowledge*. Basic, New York.
Goffman, E. (1961) *Asylums*. Penguin, Harmondsworth.
Goodman, N. (1978) *Ways of Worldmaking*. Harvester, Hassocks.
Ingold, T. (ed.) (1997) *Key Debates in Anthropology*. Routledge, London.
Larkin, P. (1990) *Collected Poems*. Faber/Marvell, London.
Leach, E. R. (1982) *Social Anthropology*. Fontana, London.
Leach, E. R. (1984) Glimpses of the unmentionable in the history of British social anthropology. *Annual Review of Anthropology* **13**, 1–23.
Leach, E. R. (1989) Writing anthropology: a review of Geertz's *Works and Lives*. *American Ethnologist* **16**(1), 137–141.
Louch, A. (1966) *Explanation and Human Action*. Blackwell, Oxford.
Needham, R. (1978) *Primordial Characters*. University of Virginia Press, Charlottesville, VA.
Nietzsche, F. (1911) On truth and falsity in their ultramoral sense (1873). In *Early Greek Philosophy, and Other Essays*. Foulis, London.
Prigogine, I. (1989) The philosophy of instability. *Futures* August, 396–400.

Rapport, N. J. (1994) *The Prose and the Passion. Anthropology, Literature and the Writing of E. M. Forster*. Manchester University Press, Manchester.

Rapport, N. J. (1997a) Opposing the motion that 'Cultural studies will be the death of anthropology', Group for Debates in Anthropological Theory, Department of Social Anthropology, University of Manchester.

Rapport, N. J. (1997b) *Transcendent Individual: Towards a Liberal and Literary Anthropology*. Routledge, London.

Rapport, N. J. (2000) Writing on the body: the poetic life-story of Philip Larkin. *Anthropology and Medicine* **7**(1), 39–62.

Rapport, N. J. (2002) The computer as a focus of inattention: five scenarios concerning hospital porters. In H. Wulff & C. Garsten (eds) *New Technologies at Work*. Berg, Oxford.

Rapport, N. J. (2003) *I am Dynamite: An Alternative Anthropology of Power*. Routledge, London.

Rapport, N., Dawson, A. (1998) Home and movement: a polemic. In N. Rapport & A. Dawson (eds) *Migrants of Identity. Perceptions of Home in a World of Movement*. Berg, Oxford.

Wagner, R. (1977) Culture as creativity. In J. Dolgin, D. Kemnitzer & D. Schneider (eds) *Symbolic Anthropology*. Columbia University Press, New York.

Watson, L., Watson-Franke, M.-B. (1985) *Interpreting Life-Histories*. Rutgers University Press, New Brunswick.

Weiner, J. (1995) Anthropologists, historians and the secret of social knowledge. *Anthropology Today* **11**(5), 3–7.

Wiener, N. (1949) *Cybernetics*. John Wiley & Sons, New York.

10 Philosophy, Nursing and the Nature of Evidence

P. ANNE SCOTT

School of Nursing, Dublin City University, Ireland

INTRODUCTION

The use of philosophical inquiry or philosophical analysis is quite a recent phenomenon in the nursing literature (Kikuchi & Simmons 1992). It seems relevant therefore to spend a short time considering what philosophical analysis looks like and what some of its uses in nursing might be. Simply put, philosophical analysis involves the following:

- the analysis of concepts – such as 'care', 'holism', 'evidence', 'advocacy';
- the uncovering of assumptions;
- analysis of lines of reasoning;
- the determination of what would count as good reasons in specific situations;
- a consideration of the bases, development and structure of arguments.

It can be seen that attention to these elements in thinking and/or writing about an issue should lead to greater clarity, consistency and soundness in one's thinking and writing. For example, the position being taken in this chapter is that attention to the above elements would make our nursing scholarship and research sounder and more coherent. The hope is that this would also lead to sounder, more coherent practice.

Historically, a number of nursing authors have used the term 'philosophy of nursing' to refer to a broad vision of nursing in terms of its means and ends (Marriner-Tomcy 1994, p. 74) or indeed more explicitly as a belief system (Gortner 1990; Salsberry 1995). However, I suggest that nursing does not need to acquire or adopt a broad vision or a belief system from philosophy. Many would suggest that nursing's religious and military roots already equip it with such sets of values and beliefs in sufficient measure. Our codes of conduct in their various guises attempt to articulate the value base of the profession. Professional socialisation processes also work to do something similar in a more covert manner – that does not always cohere with our code of conduct.

Interdisciplinary Research: Diverse Approaches in Science, Technology, Health and Society.
Edited by J. Atkinson and M. Crowe.
Copyright © 2006 by John Wiley & Sons, Ltd.

I suggest that what nursing does need from philosophy – or at least what nursing could greatly benefit from – is an ethos and tools to challenge, develop, modify, change and hone the clarity and implications of the values articulated in our codes and so forth. In other words, the tools of philosophy could help nurse scholars articulate, with greater clarity, what we claim as central to clinical nursing practice. They could also assist us to consider the implications of these claims for the profession, individual practitioners and for patient care. Thus I suggest that nurses need at least a passing acquaintance with some of the skills of philosophers, such as:

- conceptual analysis;
- the ability to identify and clarify underlying assumptions;
- argumentation.

A pertinent example where such skills would be very useful to the profession, and would be influential in patient care, is the issue of 'evidence', as used in the notion of 'evidence-based practice'. It seems timely to consider what is meant by 'evidence' in this context. We might also usefully inquire regarding the nature of the assumptions underlying the evidence-based practice movement.

THE NOTION OF EVIDENCE

What is 'evidence'? In normal parlance 'evidence' is some thing X – some statement, thing, situation and so forth – that provides support for, confidence in, or grounds for acceptance of statement, conclusion Y. We look for evidence in many of our normal daily activities, from driving our cars (what side of the road should we drive on, are the traffic lights working?) to eating our meals (is this a good place to eat, is this food good for me?). There is nothing magical about the notion of evidence. It is part of our daily existence. However, what is important is to consider how one determines what to choose as evidence from all the plethora of details, facts and information that we come across in our daily and professional lives. How does one determine what is evidence and what is not?

This brings us on to our first point of clarification. When we speak of evidence we speak of *evidence for something*. There is not evidence *per se*. The notion of evidence must be directed at an object – *evidence for X* is evidence in relation to some specified issue or situation. Thus, as Downie and Macnaughton (2000) suggest, the determination of information or facts as evidence assumes that this information and/or fact(s) has been submitted to the scrutiny of an assessor – a human being or group of human beings with particular backgrounds, experience and/or expertise that qualifies them to determine that X is evidence in support of Y. This individual or group determines what the value, significance or weight of X is, as evidence in support of or contraindication of Y. Thus three things become clear about the notion of evidence: first, it is normative (X is being seen as valuable or not valuable information or facts with regard to situation Y); second, the notion of evidence is dependent on the notion of judgement. In other words the assessor(s) is making value judgements regarding (a) whether X is evidence in the first instance and (b) what the worth of so-called evidence X is in relation to particular issue or situation Y. This would of course suggest, thirdly, that the idea of the totally 'objective' nature of evidence may be called into serious question.

> From one point of view, evidence is really just information, but it is a certain kind of information in that it relates to a specific conclusion. We do not just say 'The evidence', we say, 'This is evidence for something or that something is the case.' Information and data can be about something but they do not suggest that we must draw any conclusion from them.
> ... First the facts have to be relevant to the case and they must be relevant in a particular way – i.e. in that they are facts that contribute to a specific hypothesis relating to the case.
> ... Second, there must be some assessment of the extent to which these facts suggest this conclusion. (How relevant they are.)
> ... The third and final point about handling of facts as evidence is that they must be submitted to the judgement of an assessor. (Downie & Macnaughton 2000, pp. 8–9)

Downie and Macnaughton go on:

> This point needs to be stressed ... as it is an important point of distinction between facts and evidence. Facts or data can be accepted without recourse to judgement but facts as evidence necessarily involves judgement. The concept of evidence is therefore parasitic on the concept of judgement. Now the concept of judgement is normative in the sense that to prioritise certain facts as the important ones, or it is claiming that certain facts amount to good evidence. ... We can therefore say that the concept of evidence (which relies on judgement) must also be normative. In other words, the conclusion that some facts or pieces of data constitute 'evidence' for something is not arrived at through an entirely objective process; it depends on some individual or group evaluation. (Downie & Macnaughton 2000, p. 10)

This seems to be an incredibly important insight for nurses and doctors to grasp and ponder. I suggest that the conception of evidence, as used in the evidence-based medicine and evidence-based practice literature, has taken on some form of magical, unchallengeable identity, based apparently on the assumed objectivity of the nature of 'evidence' *per se*. A further problem, I suggest, with the notion of evidence as used in this literature is that it is exceedingly narrow in focus and, if embraced fully and exclusively, denigrates or ignores entirely large aspects of clinical practice that are not amenable to scientific investigation or measurement.

Important questions to ask at this point are:

- What is the nature of nursing (or medicine)?
- What is the practice's central focus?

In the light of answers to the former two questions, further questions might be:

- What could be deemed the types or elements of practice that require evidence?
- What might this kind of evidence look like?

Borrowing Downie and Macnaughton's definition – what sources of information should the practitioner draw on, in order to have information/facts that will be judged by an assessor as relevant to a specific hypothesis(es)? What sources of information must the practitioner draw on in order, in other words, to have evidence on which to base practice?

However, before moving on to consider these issues it also needs to be noted that frequently in the nursing literature the notion of evidence-based practice is used synonymously with 'research-based practice'. This seems problematic as the notions of evidence and research are not synonymous – i.e. something could be deemed to count as evidence for X, yet not be the product of any formalised research activity. Estabrooks (1998, p. 16), for example, suggests that:

> research utilization is a subset of evidence-based practice and that the term *evidence-based practice* ought to encompass a much broader range of evidence than the findings of scientific research.

Downie and Macnaughton (2000) would take a very similar stance, indicating that of the three types of 'scientific' research engaged in, in medical science, only a small proportion of this research was of relevance to clinical medical practice. The three types of medical scientific research engaged in, as identified by Downie and Macnaughton, are:

1. Systematic investigation and knowledge of the systems of the body and their pathology.
2. Descriptive studies, including qualitative studies, exploring clinician and patient behaviour and their interaction.
3. Randomised, controlled trials (RCTs).

Surely this type of scientific work is important as a basis for medical and nursing practice? Why is it suggested that this in fact forms the basis for only a small amount of practice? Downie and Macnaughton, for example, suggest that clinical practice extends far beyond the information provided by the above three types of medical research. They focus on the narrative nature of medical practice and the importance of clinical experience in clinical judgement and decision making.

Even from the above listing, the accuracy of Downie and Macnaughton's claims appears to hold face validity. Thus clinicians need a broader conception of the type of evidence that is of value in clinical practice. The corollary to this would be, as indicated above, that deeper, more sustained attention needed to be given to the nature of clinical practice and what might sensibly be deemed as relevant in terms of evidence to support and develop good practice and to dissipate unsafe, ineffective practice.

EVIDENCE-BASED MEDICINE

The notion of 'evidence-based practice' had grown out of the evidence-based medicine (EBM) movement of the early 1990s. However, Sackett et al. (1996, p. 71) suggest that the philosophical origins of evidence-based medicine date back to mid-nineteenth-century France.

Rosenberg and Donald (1995, pp. 1123–1125) suggest that 'EBM is the process of systematically finding, appraising and using contemporaneous research findings as the basis for clinical decisions ... The evidence will not automatically dictate patient care but will provide the factual basis on which decisions can be made, taking all aspects of patient care into consideration.'

Kitson (1997), looking specifically at nursing and where it fits into the evidence-based movement, in a guarded and carefully worded article identifies what she terms three major assumptions of EBM:

- clinicians directly involved in delivering patient care influence, either positively or negatively, patient outcomes;
- clinicians assume full responsibility for their practice;
- drawing on and contributing to a body of knowledge elucidates best evidence and optimum effectiveness.

Kitson goes on to warn nurses thus: 'By trying to counter outmoded views of [nursing] nurses may embrace the evidence-based movement without fully understanding the rules. And as written at the moment, the rules are about medical diagnosis, single clinical interventions, RCTs and meta-analysis. It is acknowledged that there is a limit to nursing evidence conforming to these criteria. What must not happen is that nurses are then excluded from the movement because their research is too poor or insufficient in rigor or size' (p. 38). Kitson goes on:

> What the EBM and CE movement have done is to help nursing demonstrate its contribution to patient care. This will continue if EBM and CE can acknowledge the characteristics of nursing which call for a broader methodological base upon which to evaluate evidence.

I think Kitson makes a number of important points here but apparently she does not challenge the concept of evidence used.

What is meant by 'evidence' in this context? It seems quite clear that Sackett et al. (1996) and Rosenberg and Donald (1995), and indeed Kitson, to a degree assume that evidence means scientific evidence.

This is of course only accurate if one equates evidence with scientific results as such. One thing that a philosophical approach may do is help to challenge and clarify the conceptualisation and thus the definition of evidence used – both in clinical practice and in our literature.

Four interesting assumptions appear to be made in the evidence-based practice literature:

1. All clinical practice is amenable to the acquisition of a scientific (ultimately based on RCTs) evidence (research) base.
2. Once this scientific evidence base is developed it can and will be adopted by clinicians in their everyday practice.
3. The adoption of this scientific evidence base will ensure excellent clinical practice.
4. Excellent clinical practice means excellent patient care, including good patient outcomes.

The reasonableness of any or all of these assumptions of course depends on the answers one generates to the questions posed above. Once again these questions are:

- What is the nature of nursing (or medical) practice?
- What is the practice's central focus?

In the light of answers to the former two questions, further questions might be:

- What could be deemed the types or elements of practice that require evidence?
- What might this kind of evidence look like – what sources of information should the practitioner draw on?

WHAT IS THE NATURE OF NURSING PRACTICE?

Much has been written over the past century regarding nursing and medical practice. In the latter part of the twentieth century, for example, the importance of the moral dimension of nursing practice and the problem of the invisibility of nursing are both highlighted in our literature. Nursing has been variously described as a caring profession (Benner & Wrubel 1989), moral action (Atkinson 1997), containing a significant moral dimension (Griffin 1980; Sarvimaki 1995; Scott 1997), having a moral goal (Scott 1995) and as being a moral practice or enterprise (Nortvedt 1998).

Occupations may be defined by the aim (e.g. farming), the role (a judge), the skill (a musician) or by all three – for example, a teacher. I suggest nursing or medicine can also be described by all three: role, skill and aim. Nursing is a socially recognised and prescribed role; it is also the case that certain skills must be acquired by the practitioner before he/she is registered and enabled to use the title 'nurse' (Downie 1971). Nursing can also be seen to have an aim – the provision of appropriate care for those who are ill or in need of nursing care.

Is nursing then a practice rooted in moral concerns? It may be useful to consider the motivation to nurse, the duties and obligations of the role and the goal or aim of nursing practice. Regarding motivation to nurse, this seems quite mixed: nursing has traditionally been an acceptable female profession; many enter nursing seeking a socially respected job, and the possibility of continuous employment. There are, of course, motivations that stem directly from idealism and a wish to be of service. There is also, in some societies, a status issue.

The duties and obligations of the role of nurse are largely socially determined and supported through licence to practise. Some of these duties are moral duties but some do not seem to have salient moral content – for example the payment of the Nursing and Midwifery Council or An Bórd Altranais (Irish Nursing Board) registration fee at the appointed time. I think the jury is out on the notion that nursing is entirely rooted in moral concerns – though there are a number of authors who claim this of both nursing and medicine (Downie 1964).

Thus, I do not want to support the strong claim that nursing is a moral enterprise or a moral practice as such. However, it does seem perfectly possible to support the weaker claim that nursing has a significant moral element, indeed perhaps even a moral goal. This is the case for a number of reasons.

In the first place it is clear that many nursing activities do have a direct impact on a person/patient. And that impact is to the benefit or detriment of that person, for example, careless or incompetent care which leads to injury, pressure sore development, lack of recognition of significant postoperative complications or malnutrition.

We also know of many counter-examples, such as that described by Oakley (1993), of the young nurse whom the patient perceives as having a profound impact on his or her care – for example, the nurse who sits and listens, sensitively and intelligently, to a patient's concerns and then provides the needed information and support. The following quotation from the medical sociologist Anne Oakley may help to put some of this in context and also highlights to some extent the identified problem of nursing's invisibility.

Oakley (1993) stated that having spent over twenty years as a medical sociologist, she had no clear idea what nurses did until she herself became a patient:

A young nurse came into the room to fetch the remains of my lunch, and she saw that I was distressed. Instead of taking my lunch tray away, or offering me drugs for the pain I was in, she sat down on my bed and held my hand and talked to me. I told her how I felt, and after a while she went away and read my notes, then came back and told me everything that was in them, and that in her, of course unmedical view, I would probably be alright. She stayed with me for nearly an hour, which she should not have done. I was radioactive and no-one was meant to spend any longer than ten minutes at a time with me. She was also presumably not supposed to tell me what was in my case notes, so she was breaking at least two sets of rules. I never saw this nurse again after I left hospital, but I would like her to know that she was important to my survival. (Oakley 1993, pp. 39–40)

In the second place, as illustrated in the above quotation, the activity of nursing is directed at an aim. I would argue that this aim or goal, patient comfort or well being, is clearly a moral aim or goal, having as it does the essential element of some notion of the good for a person/patient as human being.

For example, Edwards (1998, p. 399) describes the end of nursing as 'to promote health or well-being'. This notion of the good for a human being and of the duty of nurses to promote this type of end is commonly discussed in our ethics literature – for example Levine (1977), Gadow (1980), Bandman and Bandman (1995) and Bergum (1994). It is also of course articulated in our Code of Professional Conduct (An Bórd Altranais 2000).

WHAT IS THE CENTRAL FOCUS OF NURSING?

It seems to me very hard to argue against the notion that the role of nurse or doctor primarily exists, and is sanctioned by society, to do people good. This good is not in terms of increasing their financial status or their attractiveness to the job market, but to do people good through caring for their health, and thus to do people good as human beings. In the latter part of the twentieth and early twenty-first centuries this focus on doing people good, from a health care perspective, has been articulated in individualistic terms with the emphasis being placed on individual difference and uniqueness, such as can be found in the rhetoric surrounding notions of individualised patient care or personalised treatment (Alexander et al. 2000, p. 959; European Charter of Patients' Rights 2002).

Much of the concern here appears to be to ensure that the importance of the individual and individual difference is recognised and respected during the receipt of nursing and health care. This concern with the individual and recognition of the need to translate from or mediate general laws, rules and principles to the context of the individual is also recognised in some medical literature.

In the early 1990s Montgomery Hunter, for example, described medical practice thus:

The practice of medicine is an interpretative activity. It is the art of adjusting scientific abstractions to the individual case. The details of individual maladies are made sense of and treatment undertaken in the light of the principles of biological sciences.

Yet medicine's focus is the individual patient – fitting general principles to the individual case – means that the knowledge possessed by clinicians is narratively constructed and transmitted. How else can the individual be known? (Montgomery Hunter 1991)

She goes on:

Medicine is not science. Instead, it is a rational, science-using, inter-level interpretive activity undertaken for the care of a sick person.

As an interpretive activity turned towards an endless succession of individuals, it takes the patient as its text and seeks to understand his or her malady in the light of current biological, epistemological and psychological knowledge. (Montgomery Hunter 1991)

The patient–practitioner encounter is between and among individuals who certainly share the biology of body systems and probably similar physiology and patho-physiological processes. However, there are also aspects of nursing and medical practice that are determined by the unique, the individual. Downie and Macnaughton suggest the following:

medicine is an art in the following senses: it involves the weighing of evidence in individual cases, the interpretation of the patient anecdotes and other features of the consultation: the exercise of skills, including communication skills in a manner appropriate to the individual case, and leading to the obtaining of informed consent. The common thread in this, which justifies the use of the term 'art' is that there can be no rules to direct the doctor. Even 'guidelines', a fashionable idea of ruling bodies in medicine, require interpretation in individual cases. A good doctor is like a good musician: both require a basic technique and both must apply that technique to suit the occasion. In other words, in the clinical situation judgement is again central. (Downie & Macnaughton 2000, p. 71)

SOME RECENT WORK EXPLORING THE FOCUS AND CONTENT OF NURSING PRACTICE

A number of exploratory descriptive studies, using mainly qualitative methods and/or small samples have recently appeared in the literature (Bowman 1995; Buller & Butterworth 2001; Cowman et al. 1997; Dowding et al. 2001; Jinks & Hope 2000). The consistent theme in these studies is the complex and multi-faceted nature of contemporary nursing practice. For example, Dowding et al. (2001) found that staff nurses working in medical and surgical contexts spent significant proportions of their time in communication with various persons, from patients and relatives, to nurses, doctors and other co-workers. On average the nurses observed spent 37.5% of their time communicating (verbally either on the telephone or face-to-face) (mean 134.9, range 0–258). These studies also indicate that various proportions of a nurse's time are spent supporting patients from both physical and psychosocial perspectives, in direct and indirect care activities, collecting information, in administration and in patient/relative and student education, among other activities (Buller & Butterworth 2001; Cowman et al. 1997; Dowding et al. 2001; Jinks & Hope

2000). Figure 10.1 presents my own diagrammatic representation of the domains of nursing practice as outlined by Buller and Butterworth (2001).

From this diagrammatic summary and from the above brief taste of findings of recent studies exploring the nature and context of contemporary nursing practice, it can be seen that practice is multifaceted. The practitioner is socialised to the professional practice ethos (Holm 1997; Melia 1987). This socialisation process attempts to instil certain values and perceptions regarding that which is important and that which is less so or not at all. As a result of this socialisation process, the practitioner, and thus the person of the practitioner, is being formed in a certain manner. The person, as practitioner, is required to be a particular type of person – caring, sensitive, competent, compassionate (see Niven & Scott 2003; Pellegrino 1979; Pellegrino & Thomasma 1993; Scott 1995, 2000) and so forth. These personal characteristics, it is argued, shape and strongly influence the quality of the practitioner's practice and thus the quality of patient care (Niven & Scott 2003; Nortvedt 1998, 2001; Pellegrino 1979; Pellegrino & Thomasma 1993; Scott 2000). The practitioner is also required to draw on a variety of sources of knowledge and information in order to inform her/himself for effective clinical practice. Such sources range from the biological and chemical sciences, through human psychology, sociology, professional ethics, theories of management, administration, education, to current thinking on skilled practice in clinical assessment, therapeutic intervention, and evaluation of clinical outcomes.

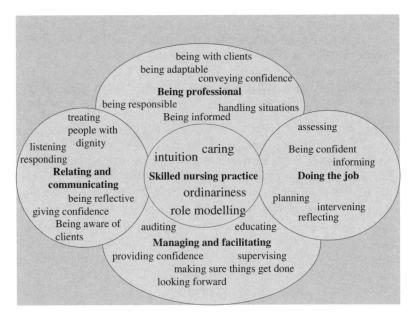

Figure 10.1. The domains of nursing practice. (Adapted from Buller & Butterworth 2001).

IS EVIDENCE REQUIRED?

Given the complexity of current nursing practice, and the potential detrimental effects of that practice on patient care, should there not be some sort of coherent evidence base to practice? It seems that the answer must be 'Yes, appropriate, relevant information and, where they exist/are available, facts are required to support effective clinical practice'. What determines that such information and/or facts is evidence? The appraisal by the practising clinician, that (a) this information and these facts are relevant to this patient case, and (b) that the material is sufficiently relevant to count as evidence for state X, diagnosis Y, explanation of an identified problem – such as non-response to treatment, non-compliance and so forth. However, given the nature and content of nursing practice (see, for example, the quotation from Oakley and the finding of Buller and Butterworth reported above), together with the possibility that the practitioner is required to have certain personal characteristics, it would seem that the 'evidence' required to form an appropriate base for practice can only sensibly be conceived of broadly.

Nurses observe, assess and intervene therapeutically (from both the physical and psychological/mental perspectives) with individual patients. They coordinate, facilitate, communicate, administer, collect information, record, remind, report, cajole, coerce, support, educate and reassure. All these activities should be based on relevant information and facts (*evidence*) when and where these are available. Nurses also engage in a number of so-called 'non-nursing' activities, at least some of which have definite nursing intent. For example, a nurse may go and tidy a patient's locker in order to have a legitimate excuse for spending some time observing or talking with a patient she/he is concerned about.

Is evidence required for all these various activities? What kind of evidence might be required? Is it all evidence of the same type? For example, in interacting supportively with a patient the nurse surely does look for evidence of patient state. She attends to a variety of important cues: a word, a glance, a measurement, a colour, a reaction, a response; she attends to non-verbal as well as verbal cues. She processes patient statements, claims, requests for information, complaints. She also needs to understand basic anatomy, physiology and patho-physiological reactions, basic drug effects, interactions, side effects, expected and unusual psychological and emotional reactions, and to assess, monitor and evaluate patient state in relation to these. What makes any of this information count as evidence? The clinician is 'tuned in' to the patient, attends to speech, colour, facial expression, behaviour. Oakley's nurse, described above, recognised her patient's distress. The clinician in the light of her professional educational background, previous clinical experience with patients having similar problems/responses and her knowledge of this particular patient interprets such cues. Such interpretations, borne from a background of professional knowledge and experience, provide the evidence or otherwise of the need for the nurse to intervene. Similarly blood tests, X-ray results and patient interviews are interpreted by the clinician. This interpretive activity is part of the process during which the various pieces of information acquired are deemed useful, relevant, irrelevant, of high priority to check out or to look for other corroborating confirming detail and so on. As suggested above, this activity is like putting pieces of a jigsaw puzzle together – or, as Downie and Macnaughton (2000) suggest, like the activities of a detective during an investigation. It is – and, given human variation, in fact it must be – the practitioner who determines what is the relevant information/facts in this particular patient case. Thus it is the practitioner who determines what is to count as evidence. What counts as evidence is not likely to be static from patient to patient. What counts as evidence is in fact likely to vary with the particular patient situation, skills demand or task in hand. Thus in order to determine what kinds of evidence are required for evidence-based practice, a detailed understanding of the elements, focus and aims of clinical nursing practice is required.

The nurse needs to coordinate this patient's care: to gather the required information, to ensure the patient is seen/examined by medical staff and any other members of the health care team deemed necessary – for example, the physiotherapist, occupational therapist, dietician, chaplain and so forth. The nurse needs to process follow-up referrals, and ensure the appropriate X-ray and blood tests are carried out and reports received in a timely fashion. She needs to see that the patient is in the correct ward at the correct time – which may involve fielding the bed manager or indeed the relevant medical consultant. Conversing with relatives may not only throw useful light on current patient condition, but also on the need for appropriate education and support of both patient and relative, and on the necessary discharge plans required for this particular patient.

WHAT IS THE NATURE OF THE EVIDENCE REQUIRED?

What seems to emerge, as suggested above, is a kind of jigsaw puzzle. When staff begin patient care, neither the picture nor the desired specific outcome is clear. During the assessment and time spent with the patient, both of these become increasingly clear, assuming appropriate interaction with health care staff. As the former two elements become clearer the required health care and nursing interventions also begin to be identified. Such identification in turn leads to assessment and evaluations of the effects of the interventions; and to continuance, modification, change or termination of the interventions. This latter process, no less than the initial information gathering and picture building can be a painstaking, inch-by-inch type activity. General principles may suggest X. However, the particularities of this patient and context may actually require X_1 or A.

A problem for nursing and for medicine, in terms of appropriate practice and an appropriate evidence base for practice, is that we are forced daily to deal with both the general and the particular; and to determine, with each clinical interaction, how the balance between them is to be set. A further problem is the centrality of meaning in human as against physical science. Rocks do not spend time attempting to interpret the meaning behind their particular existence or the position of their neighbouring rock. Rocks simply are. Human beings are and have various theories regarding why this is so – from a biological, social and personal perspective. As human beings we also spend our lives interpreting events and ascribing meaning to these events – including our illnesses and our recovery or otherwise. This introduces a number of complexities into the issue of the required evidence base for clinical health care/nursing practice. Perhaps for this reason, as Downie and Macnaughton (2000) suggest, much of clinical practice is more akin to detective work than it is to science – piecing the puzzle together is the only effective way to reach an appropriate and effective conclusion, from the perspective of either the patient or indeed the practitioner.

Nurses and doctors normally are responsible for a group of patients rather than one individual patient and this also needs to be recognised. Thus, for example, from a resourcing perspective the needs of the collective may require to be identified and weighted against the individual. However, as the psychologist Gordon Allport (1955) reminds us, every man is like all other men, like some other men, like no other man – presumably this goes for women also. From the perspective of the patient, his/her illness is very particular, very personal. Sometimes, no doubt, it is useful and reassuring to discover that more than oneself is suffering, indeed suffering from X and having reaction Y. Nonetheless, there will be elements of the illness, the treatment or the context that are specific to the person. Thus there are shared and unique elements of each jigsaw puzzle that the practitioner must be equipped to identify and deal with. Each specific situation must be considered, interpreted, diagnosed, treated and cared for.

Thus it would seem that the nurse draws on evidence in providing appropriate nursing care for a patient; in fact she/he draws on a lot of different kinds of evidence. Thus the answer to question number three above is 'A number of different elements of nursing practice require evidence for effective practice'. The answer to question number four above is 'This evidence has a variety of sources' – from facial expression (interpreted via pattern recognition), through evidence of effective administration (from a variety of feedback mechanisms) to biological evidence such as skin colour and temperature readings. Not all of the evidence required for effective nursing practice is scientific in nature. In fact science and scientific evidence have an important but limited role in clinical practice and the notion of evidence within the context of evidence-based practice needs to be broadened out considerably if it is to benefit patients and maintain the integrity of both nursing and medicine.

CONCLUSION

Ideals of practice focus on the uniqueness of the individual. Research on activities and decision making in clinical practice suggest multi-skilled staff that effectively prioritise patient care needs even in the most extreme of circumstances. Staffs are constantly interrupted in care provision and need to know how to handle this, while dealing with a myriad of patient needs and negotiating the hierarchical terrain of the clinical practice context. In order to identify the evidence base for practice – in nursing or medicine – we must be clearer regarding that which the practice comprises.

Nurses spend much time scanning, interpreting, liaising, supporting. I suggest that science looks a rather too limiting evidence base to work from, when looking through the lens of clinical nursing practice. Philosophical analysis in this instance should help us become clearer on the notion of evidence, on the nature of the evidence required and on the inherently normative and non-objective nature of elements of decisions regarding what is and is not to count as evidence in any particular case.

REFERENCES

Alexander, M. F., Fawcett, J. N., Runciman, P. J. (eds) (2000) *Nursing Practice: Hospital and Home.* Churchill Livingstone, Edinburgh.

Allport, G. W. (1955) *Becoming: Basic Considerations for a Psychology of Personality.* Yale University Press, New Haven, CT.

Atkinson, J. (1997) A descriptive and evaluative study of district nursing intervention with single homeless men from a private hostel in Glasgow, PhD thesis, Glasgow Caledonian University, Glasgow.

Bandman, E. L., Bandman, B. (1995) *Nursing Ethics Through the Life Span*, 3rd edn. Prentice Hall, Englewood Cliffs, NJ.

Benner, P., Wrubel, J. (1989) *The Primacy of Caring: Stress and Coping in Health and Illness.* Addison-Wesley, Menlo Park, CA.

Bergum, V. (1994) Knowledge for ethical care. *Nursing Ethics* 1(2), 71–79.

Bowman, M. (1995) *The Professional Nurse.* Chapman & Hall, London.

Buller, S., Butterworth, T. (2001) Skilled nursing practice – a qualitative study of the elements of nursing. *International Journal of Nursing Studies* 38, 405–417.

Cowman, S., Farrelly, M., Gilheaney, P. (1997) *The Role and Function of the Psychiatric Nurse in Clinical Practice.* St Vincent's Hospital, Fairview, Dublin.

Dowding, D., Scott, P. A., Niven, K., Taylor, A., Morrison, A. (2001) Examining the interventions of nurses in acute medical and surgical units in Scotland. In N. Oud (ed.) *ACENDIO: Proceedings of the Third European Conference of the Association of Common European Nursing Diagnoses, Interventions and Outcomes, Berlin 2001* (pp. 135–136). Verlag Hans Huber, Bern.

Downie, R. S. (1964) *Government Action and Morality.* Macmillan, London.

Downie, R. S. (1971) *Roles and Values: An Introduction to Social Ethics.* Metheun, London.

Downie, R. S., Macnaughton, J. (2000) *Clinical Judgement: Evidence in Clinical Practice*. Oxford University Press, Oxford.

Edwards, S. (1998) The art of nursing: *Nursing Ethics* **5**, 393–400.

Estabrooks, C. A. (1998) Will evidence-based nursing practice make practice perfect? *Canadian Journal of Nursing Research* **30**(1), 15–36.

European Charter of Patients' Rights (2002) Available at: http://www.activecitizenship.net/health/italian_charter.pdf. Accessed 20 June 2004.

Gadow, S. (1980) Existential advocacy: philosophical foundation of nursing. In S. Spicker & S. Gadow (eds) *Nursing: Images and Ideals. Opening Dialogue with the Humanities* (pp. 79–102). Springer, New York.

Gortner, S. (1990) Nursing values and science: towards a science philosophy. *Image* **22**, 101–105.

Griffin, A. P. (1980) Philosophy and nursing. *Journal of Advanced Nursing* **5**, 261–272.

Holm, S. (1997) *Ethical Problems in Clinical Practice*. Manchester University Press, Manchester.

Jinks, A. M., Hope, P. (2000) What do nurses do? An observational survey of the activities of nurses on acute surgical and rehabilitation wards. *Journal of Nursing Management* **8**, 273–279.

Kikuchi, J., Simmons, H. (eds) (1992) *Philosophic Inquiry in Nursing*. Sage, Newbury Park, CA.

Kitson, A. (1997) Using evidence to demonstrate the place of nursing. *Nursing Standard* **11**(28), 34–39.

Levine, M. E. (1977) Nursing ethics and the ethical nurse. *American Journal of Nursing* **77**, 845–849.

Marriner-Tomey, A. (1994) *Nursing Theorists and their Work*, 3rd edn. Mosby, St Louis, MO.

Melia, K. M. (1987) *Learning and Working: The Occupational Socialisation of Nurses*. Tavistock, London.

Montgomery Hunter, K. (1991) *Doctors' Stories: The Narrative Structure of Medical Knowledge*. Princeton University Press, Princeton, NJ.

Niven, C. A., Scott, P. A. (2003) The need for accurate perception and informed judgement in determining the appropriate use of the nursing resource: hearing the patient's voice. *Nursing Philosophy* **4**, 201–210.

Nortvedt, P. (1998) Sensitive judgement: an inquiry into the foundations of nursing ethics. *Nursing Ethics* **5**, 385–392.

Nortvedt, P. (2001) Clinical sensitivity: the inseparability of ethical perceptiveness and clinical knowledge. *Scholarly Inquiry of Nursing Practice* **15**(3), 1–19.

Oakley, A. (1993) *Essays on Women, Medicine and Health*. Edinburgh University Press, Edinburgh.

Pellegrino, E. D. (1979) *Humanism and the Physician*. University of Tennessee Press, Knockville, TN.

Pellegrino, E. D., Thomasma, D. C. (1993) *The Virtues in Medical Practice*. Oxford University Press, New York.

Rosenberg, W., Donald, A. (1995) Evidence based medicine: an approach to clinical problem-solving. *British Medical Journal* **310**, 1122–1126.

Sackett, D. L., Rosenberg, W. M. C., Muir Gray, J. A., Haynes, R. B., Richardson, W. S. (1996) Evidence based medicine: what it is and what it isn't. *British Medical Journal* **312**, 71–72.

Salsberry, P. J. (1995) A philosophy of nursing: what is it and what is it not? In J. Kikuchi & H. Simmons (eds) *Developing a Philosophy of Nursing*. Sage, Newbury Park, CA.

Sarvimaki, A. (1995) Knowledge in interactive practice disciplines. Stockholm University, College of Health Science, Unit for Research and Development, Stockholm.

Scott, P. A. (1995) Care, attention and imaginative identification in nursing practice. *Journal of Advanced Nursing* **21**, 1196–1200.

Scott, P. A. (1997) Imagination in practice. *Journal of Medical Ethics* **23**(1), 45–50.

Scott, P. A. (2000) Emotion, moral perception and nursing practice. *Nursing Philosophy* **1**(2), 123–133.

11 Researching the Spiritual: Outcome or Process?

HARRIET MOWAT and JOHN SWINTON
Mowat Research Ltd, Aberdeen, UK and Department of Divinity and Religious Studies, Aberdeen, UK

INTRODUCTION

The purpose of the chapter is to try to tease out some of the difficulties inherent in researching a topic that has not yet been finally defined. The topic under discussion here is spiritual care giving. It considers the challenges of using an interpretive method (in particular ethnography) in a research study that is located in what is essentially a positivist paradigm of thinking. The setting is the National Health Service and the funder is the Scottish Executive. Both these organisations set great store by evidence-based practice and therefore research that can produce evidence. Both these organisations see the 'gold standard' method for deriving evidence as one that can make causal connections through statistical analysis. Both organisations highly value the ability of research to make recommendations based on these statistical causal relationships.

A real tension exists here therefore in the attempt to look at spiritual care giving. On the one hand there are the reasonable requirements of the funder to produce coherent conclusions from which policy can be derived and in which practice can be rooted. This makes the research useful and good value. On the other hand, there is the research requirement to excavate as much 'truth' about the situation of spiritual care giving as is possible in a framework that suggests the meaning and practice of spiritual care giving is 'negotiated'.

It is not just a hostile or competitive philosophical environment which challenges unfamiliar research methods but also the actual process of the research act as it is currently configured and understood by the research community. This process is very much mindful of the Research Assessment Exercise, which currently dominates the British university research world view of what is understood to be 'successful' research. Success is measured by obtaining funding that includes overheads, completion of the research task in time,

Interdisciplinary Research: Diverse Approaches in Science, Technology, Health and Society.
Edited by J. Atkinson and M. Crowe.
Copyright © 2006 by John Wiley & Sons, Ltd.

publications in highly rated journals, and national or international acclaim for the university department involved. This process often involves the use of temporary research assistants for whom the university has no continued responsibility once the research project is over and who by definition are itinerant.

This chapter refers to a recent research report co-written by the authors (Mowat & Swinton 2005). The chapter comments on the use of ethnography as part of the data collection strategy. The use of ethnography was originally a central part of the research method. The grant applicants assumed that there was no other way to capture the evolving and ever-changing nature of chaplaincy. A survey, set of questionnaires or indeed semi-structured interviews would not have been able to capture chaplaincy 'in motion'. In the event the ethnographic component of the study became troublesome for a number of epistemological and practical reasons.

A little background might be helpful.

WHY DO THE STUDY?

Chaplaincy within the National Health Service in Scotland has been and continues to be an important dimension of the drive towards a more holistic perspective on care. There is a general acceptance of the need for chaplaincy. However, when one gets down to issues of precisely what needs chaplains are actually expected to meet, things become much less clear. While there has been some important research done on chaplains in England (Mitchell 1999; Orchard 2000; Woodward 1998) to date, there has been very little research done on the nature of chaplaincy and the crucial question of what precisely it is that chaplains do. The recent implementation in Scotland of national chaplaincy guidelines (Scottish Executive 2002), which place an onus on Health Boards to address the spiritual dimensions of care, combined with the growing movement within chaplaincy that seeks to develop chaplaincy as a health care profession on a par with other health care professions, suggests there is a pressing need for the development of an evidence base that will provide concrete answers to the crucial question: what do chaplains do?

The Quality Health Care Division of the Scottish Executive funded an 18-month study exploring the role and function of the hospital chaplain within the National Health Service in Scotland. The study was carried out in 2003–2004 and involved all of the full-time hospital chaplains working for the National Health Service in Scotland.

The final report describes a process model of chaplaincy. This model emerged from engagement with chaplains over a variety of issues. It suggests that chaplaincy in Scotland is in transition. The data presented attempts to reflect, and capture, some vital insights into the role and function of the hospital chaplain. It is hoped that these insights and perspectives will enable the significance of chaplaincy for contemporary health care practices to be clearly seen. It is also hoped that the data presented will enable chaplains to reflect critically on their current practices and move towards the development of a model of professionalisation which is clearly perceived as relevant within the multidisciplinary team, but which also enables chaplains to retain their unique integrity as distinctively *spiritual* caregivers.

THE OBJECTIVES OF THE STUDY

These were:

- to build on the existing knowledge around the areas of chaplaincy, spirituality, religion and their relation to the process of health care within the Scottish National Health Service;
- to describe the current role and function of the hospital chaplain;
- to explore the various perceptions of the work of the chaplain held within the health care context;
- to identify what patients perceive as the most beneficial approaches to spiritual care and support;
- to put these findings into the context of the national guidelines on spiritual care and subsequent policy documents produced by the Health Care Trusts.

THE RESEARCH QUESTION

The guiding research question was: *what do chaplains do?* This was expressed in terms of three subsidiary questions:

- What is chaplaincy and from whose perspective?
- What is spirituality and from whose perspective?
- What is spiritual care and from whose perspective?

The spirituality guidelines (Scottish Executive 2002) reflect a general growing interest in the relationship between spirituality and health.

A NOTE ABOUT THE RISING INTEREST IN SPIRITUALITY AND HEALTH CARE

An examination of the spiritual landscape in Scotland throws up some interesting observations. In line with much of Western Europe, there is a significant decrease in adherence to traditional, formal institutional religion. The decreasing number of people regularly attending places of worship evidences this. However, while traditional religion appears to be in decline, there is a corresponding *increase* in the number of people expressing the importance of spirituality for their lives and claiming to have spiritual experiences and beliefs (Davie 1994; Hay 1990). Thus spirituality appears to have migrated from the overtly religious towards a more individualistic and subjective quest that has no necessity of a formal structure, doctrinal beliefs or an anchoring community of like-minded believers. People now want to *believe* in things spiritual, but no longer wish to *belong* to traditional religious institutions (Davie 1994; Heelas et al. 2005).

This broadening understanding of spirituality is reflected in health care settings by the increasing focus on spirituality within the literature surrounding medicine, nursing, social work and occupational therapy (Cobb & Robshaw 1998), a rising interest in complementary and alternative medicine (Austin 1998) and a developing holistic view of health and illness within which the role of chaplaincy is rapidly gaining recognition.

In an environment that values highly the role of the 'specialist', such a holistic view of health presents very particular challenges to individual professions and to the ways in which multidisciplinary teams function in practice. As medicine and health care advance in knowledge of the micro-mechanisms of the ill body, so the need for greater specialisation increases. In tension with this emphasis is the practical need expressed by people encountering illness, to be treated as whole persons who require the universal and the particular to be held in critical tension throughout their experience of illness. Within such a context spirituality becomes of foremost importance.

To provide authentic holistic, active, total care requires that attention be given to providing appropriate services that meet the *actual* needs of patients and their carers, that is, not simply the needs that health care professionals may perceive or/and assume, without reference to the wishes, desires and experiences of patients. The concept of patient-focused care is currently central to Scottish/UK Government health care policy, which stresses the importance of patient and carer views informing service developments (Scottish Executive 2001, 2003). There is evidence that suggests that patients desire to have their spiritual needs met within a health care context (Murray et al. 2004). Developing strategies to meet such expressed needs is therefore very much part of current governmental approach. Reflecting these changes in contemporary Scottish culture, comes the suggestion that spirituality and spiritual care are not optional extras for 'religious people'.

RELIGION AND HEALTH: WHAT DO WE KNOW?

In the light of these cultural changes, it is not coincidental that spirituality and religion are fast becoming recognised as a significant part of the health care research agenda, even among those more inclined towards the biomedical end of the research community spectrum (Fry 2000). The extensive research work of people such as Harold Koenig and David Larson (Koenig et al. 2001) in the

United States is indicative of the possibility of developing an evidence base to explore the relationship between religion, spirituality and health. The data from such studies is suggestive of associations between religious and spiritual observance and well-being. For example, Koenig et al. (2001) report their examination of the relationship between religion and health in about 1200 studies. They rated the quality of those studies, and on a scale from 1 (= poor) to 10 (= excellent), they found 29 they rated as 10 and 84 that were rated 9. Their conclusion (in part) was that 'in the vast majority of the cross-sectional studies and prospective cohort studies we identified, religious beliefs and practices rooted within established religious traditions were found to be consistently associated with better health and predicted better health over time' (p. 591).

Religion and spirituality have been shown to be beneficial on a number of levels and in relation to a wide variety of conditions (Larson et al. 1997). Health benefits include:

- extended life expectancy;
- lower blood pressure;
- lower rates of death from coronary artery disease;
- reduction in myocardial infarction;
- increased success in heart transplants;
- reduced serum cholesterol levels;
- reduced levels of pain in cancer sufferers;
- reduced mortality among those who attend church and worship services;
- increased longevity among the elderly;
- protection against depression and anxiety;
- reduced mortality after cardiac surgery.

While there is little research within this area done specifically on chaplaincy, a recent good example of the potential this area holds is the study by Iler et al. (2001). This reports on the effects of daily visits by a chaplain to patients with chronic obstructive pulmonary disease (COPD), and compares their health outcomes with a second group with the same diagnosis who were not visited. The results showed that, by comparison, the visited group were less anxious at discharge, their length of stay was significantly less, and their satisfaction with the hospital was significantly higher. One conclusion that might be drawn is that the support of a chaplain has a demonstrable effect on the hospitalised patient, certainly with that particular diagnosis.

THE PICTURE IN SCOTLAND

In Scotland, a succession of Ministers of Health have promoted the philosophy of patient-focused care. This refers to the recognition of the importance of meeting patients' holistic needs and the importance of inclusion and choice at a number of different levels. Part of this initiative manifested in the Patient Focus and Public Involvement Programme and the setting up of a funded unit. The Patient Involvement Programme is seen as part of the core business of each of the hospital Trusts and will be judged in similar terms to the clinical standards audit. Another vital component of the patient-focused perspective is that of *cultural competence*. This is being developed by a diversity unit, where inclusion of all and a holistic perspective are pursued.

At the same time and in response to the types of changes and developments highlighted earlier, a steering group was set up to explore what was required in terms of enabling chaplains to provide effective spiritual care. This group produced a set of guidelines for good practice in chaplaincy. This process resulted in a Health Directive Letter to all Trusts, two conferences aimed at senior Trust management, the setting up of a Chaplaincy Training Unit and the production of draft policy statements by each of the Health Boards.

The Scottish Executive has funded an initiative called *Spirited Scotland*, which offers a broad perspective on spirituality and health in Scotland. It acts as a networking point, hosts a website (www.spiritedscotland.org) and issues a newsletter. In practical terms, it has supported the development of confidence among health and social care staff to deal with spiritual issues by offering educational initiatives within the Trusts. A newly formed Centre for Spirituality, Health and Disability at the University of Aberdeen, is also pursuing a research and development agenda that promises to make a significant contribution to the area of spirituality and health care.

It is clear, then, that within Scotland there is an important movement to take health care in directions which meet the types of spiritual need that are prevalent within contemporary culture.

Within the context outlined thus far, there are some corresponding fundamental shifts taking place in both the practice and the thinking around the nature and function of chaplaincy and the meaning of health and well-being. These shifts are taking place within, and in response to, the context of the societal and political changes discussed above.

CHANGES FOR HOSPITAL CHAPLAINCY

The shifts relate to the theological and philosophical roots of chaplaincy, as well as to the texture of the care that is offered by chaplaincy under the banner of 'spiritual care'. The informed creativity of chaplaincy's response to these shifts will determine the development of chaplaincy as it moves into the challenging needs-context of twenty-first-century Scotland. It is therefore important that chaplains have the time and resources to engage critically and reflectively with these processes.

One of the main changes for chaplains in Scotland relates to the movement from being a specifically *religious* carer, to a deliverer of *spiritual* care, which is defined as distinct from care that is solely focused on religion. It will be helpful to think this through in relation to the development of the definition of the term 'chaplain'. The word *chaplain*

> refers to a clergyperson who has been commissioned by a faith group or an organisation to provide pastoral service in an institution, organisation, or governmental entity. Chaplaincy refers to the general activity performed by a chaplain, which may include crisis ministry, counselling, sacraments, worship, education, help in ethical decision-making, staff support, clergy contact and community or church co-ordination. The chaplain, ordained or otherwise, is thus seen, at least traditionally, to be the representative of a particular faith community who is sent to work within a specific setting. (Smith 1990, 136)

The traditional denominationally oriented model of chaplaincy is being challenged, not only at the bureaucratic level, but also by the spiritual changes highlighted earlier. With the general movement from religion, narrowly defined, to 'spirituality' understood as a diverse human universal, has emerged a redefinition of the spiritual positioning of chaplaincy. Chaplains now tend to refer to themselves as 'spiritual carers' rather than ministers or religious carers. Departments of 'spiritual care' are now emerging within a number of Trusts, indicating a transition from 'chaplain' as defined above, to 'spiritual carer'.

Health care chaplains are now required to think about, interpret and act upon considerably wider definitions of spiritual care than previously assumed. One of the key questions that chaplains have to tackle is the issue of what health care chaplaincy actually is in the midst of the changes and transitions that are shaping Scottish culture and health care practices.

THE STUDY DESIGN

The study utilised a qualitative study design (Robson 2002). One of the difficulties that confronts the newcomer to qualitative research methods is the wide and rather vague definitions of 'method' that tend to dominate the literature. Denzin and Lincoln (2000, p. 5) note that:

> the open ended nature of the qualitative research project leads to a perpetual resistance against attempts to impose a single umbrella-like paradigm over the entire project.

It may be helpful to think of the qualitative method as one way of *seeing* and *discovering*. John McLeod (2001) suggests that:

> At its heart, qualitative research involves doing one's utmost to map and explore the meaning of an area of human experience. . . . We live in a culture which is built on thin and superficial descriptions of experience. We can 'surf' across numerous websites, flick through television channels, listen to 'sound bites,' know ourselves

and others in the context of life-compartments . . . By contrast, good qualitative research requires an *immersion* in some aspect of social life, in an attempt to capture the wholeness of that experience, followed by an attempt to convey that understanding to others.

In essence qualitative methods render the familiar strange. It is a *descriptive* method that has an inherent rigour within the data collection and analysis and generates its own internal logic. This 'way of seeing' presupposes certain assumptions about the nature of reality. It suggests that things are going to be more complicated than they appear at the outset and that common-sense understandings of the world and the reality under scrutiny, will be challenged by the qualitative research eye.

For this study, three data collection techniques were used, all of which fall within the qualitative research paradigm. All the data was written by hand rather than tape-recorded. None of the subsequent extracts can be regarded as direct verbatim quotes. Rather they are part of the researchers' notes, combined with as much faithful interpretation as seemed appropriate. See Box 11.1.

Box 11.1. Description of data collection techniques

Telephone interviews (1)

Interviews of 44 full-time health care chaplains in Scotland. Use of a four-item structure to guide the interview:

- personal journey into chaplaincy – who is the chaplain?
- typical day of the chaplain;
- working arrangements within the Trust;
- the nature and development of chaplaincy.

Case studies

Observation, interviews and informal discussions with chaplains, patients, staff and family members in three chaplaincy sites. Sites were chosen for their variety and geographical spread. Sixteen characteristics/descriptors were identified from the interview data and these were given scores for each chaplaincy site. Five sites were initially chosen and three were finally used.

Ethical permission was gained for the observation case studies. This took a very long time. This project was one of the first to use the new system, which involved more paper work, more screening bodies and uncertain protocols.

Finally, it was decided to look at three sites and re-interview all the chaplains. The re-interview was not in the original protocol but was indicated by the content and flow of the research.

Telephone interviews (2)

Second set of interviews with full-time chaplains pursuing themes derived from telephone interviews (1) and observational data.
  Themes pursued:

- leadership;
- professionalisation;
- spiritual needs of patients;
- spiritual needs of chaplains;
- religious and spiritual care;
- spiritual correctness;
- teamworking;
- working in institutions.

As can be seen, the balance of research methods changed as the research task was embarked upon.

THE STORY OF THE RESEARCH PROCESS

NEGOTIATING A METHOD BETWEEN DISCIPLINES

The grant applicants were both full-time senior academics at the time of writing the proposal. One of the applicants (Professor John Swinton) is a practical theologian by background with a well-established research tradition within theology. The other (Dr Harriet Mowat) is a gerontologist with expertise in qualitative research methods and knowledge of health services research. The first task was to discover a method that both the applicants could understand and value. This was not particularly difficult, given the growing association between practical theology and qualitative methods (Browning 1983; Swinton & Mowat 2005). The original idea was to make central the ethnographic method. As Amanda Coffey (1999, p. 2) notes, the social research methods literature is now rich with advice texts and this has 'helped to establish qualitative methods and ethnographic fieldwork as cross/interdisciplinary and "respectable"'. The choice of method was also stimulated by discussion with other colleagues who had carried out ethnographies, and the authors' own experience of participant-observation over a long period of time. This reinforced the conviction that 'just asking' was not going to yield the complexities of how spiritual need was constructed and met within a changing worldview of religion and spirituality. The grant applicants were aware, however, that ethnography has become a subject for heated debate among methodologists.

TACKLING THE EVOLVING UNDERSTANDING OF ETHNOGRAPHIC STUDY

Ethnography has its roots in anthropological enquiry and essentially attempts to understand the situation under study from the point of view of the participants by living as one of the participants. It gets below the taken-for-granted structures within the social setting and, as noted earlier, renders the familiar strange (Dowie 2002). The ethnography asks questions about structure and negotiated meaning through observation and familiarity. Early anthropologists found this style of study yielded deep and complex meaning structures and there was little difficulty with writing up these studies from the perspective of the absorbed ethnographer. By that we mean that at the early stage of ethnography the idea that the ethnographer themselves might influence the interpretation of the data was less explored. However, recently the whole issue of interpretation of data and negotiation of realities has rendered ethnographic work and the idea of representation of others' positions as problematic (Goodall 2000). This view can be taken to extremes, where the researcher/ethnographer can only present a view or a position to the reader as one position among many and in one moment in time. The extension of this is that no one can say anything about how anybody else might think or feel or act because these actions and thoughts are temporary, and entirely the province of the thinker and actor. The observations themselves become negotiated. The observer even as participant has no ability (or right) to interpret – or at least only from their own point of view. It is therefore the observer's perspective not the participant's that is represented. In terms of the chaplains study, this would mean that the ethnographer could only say what he/she thought and saw and how he/she interpreted the difference between spiritual and religious need, not how the chaplains or patients interpreted these differences.

THE UNREALISTIC TIMESCALE

There were also some practical considerations. The study was intended to be completed within 18 months and it was originally proposed that six ethnographies be carried out with which comparisons could be made. Not withstanding the philosophical difficulties of ethnography, the practical difficulties of collecting data, analysing it and writing it up in six different settings became obvious almost as the ink dried on the paper! Almost immediately we had two major difficulties with the method: first, the philosophical and epistemological problems of ethnographic representation, and, second, the practical problems of time and resource.

THE GRANT APPLICANT AND RESEARCHER RELATIONSHIP

Once the money was granted we advertised for a research assistant. It is customary of course, and it is expected, that grant holders who have applied for funding and included a research salary in the application will not gather the lion's share of the data. Grant holders act, on the whole, as managers and supervisors.

It became obvious that we were not going to find someone with the necessary extremely sophisticated ethnographic skills and that we had in fact written the proposal for ourselves rather than for a researcher. This is no doubt a very common mistake. While the method was entirely appropriate the idea that we could employ someone for an 18-month short-term contract to do this work was hopeful to say the least.

We revised the method based on what we could reasonably deliver. We decided that a more manageable approach was to interview all the chaplains over the telephone using an open-ended structure, and, using the themes that emerged from these interviews, we would identify the ethnography sites. This would be slightly more structured – thus producing more philosophical problems – but reducing data overload and fatigue problems.

In the event, the study produced three ethnographies employing two researchers. Even so the data was difficult to corral in a way that could really do justice to the effort put in to the field work so it was decided to re-interview the chaplains at the end of the study, again over the phone, this time with a series of headings which had emerged from and been the object of observation in the field work.

The data collection techniques still seemed coherent but the ethnographic aspirations were very much tempered, probably ultimately to the advantage of the study.

A further problem with the ethnographic aspirations was that of ethics.

ETHICAL PERMISSION

Gaining ethical permission to carry out ethnographic research in the National Health Service was not the easiest of tasks.

Our study presented itself for ethical permission just as the system was changing and research governance was beefing up its profile. This meant that we were required to observe the multi-centre research ethics committee (MREC) procedures because we wanted to have permission to visit more than three sites. This lengthy form is aimed at the 'gold standard' research method, the clinical trial, and its wording tends to favour this kind of approach. Letters of permission seeking, information sheets and, in particular, details of any questions to be asked were all sought. The latter was the most problematic.

It goes without saying that knowing precisely what questions would be asked prior to the ethnography negates and renders meaningless the ethnographic process. Thus a compromise between the requirements of the form and the need for ethical permission to proceed, and the need to maintain the integrity of the method, became a challenge.

The compromise was to identify the themes that would guide the ethnography. At this stage we started talking about a case study rather than an ethnography. A case study is not a method but a unit of analysis. We refocused our attention on the unit of analysis – the chaplain – and used different data collection techniques – interview, informal interview, observation, written documents – to try to answer the question *What do chaplains do?*

GETTING AT THE 'TRUTH'

In this study there is a dual challenge in getting at the 'truth' (Swinton & Mowat, 2005). The interpretive research paradigm assumes that the truth is relative and largely a social negotiation between participants. The research task is to unearth the negotiations. However, the subject matter of the nature of spirituality, faith and belief is in the views of strong believers a truth that is undeniable. Sometimes this truth is referenced to Biblical scriptures. The response 'we know that this is so because God tells us this in the Bible' is a very far cry from the sociological interpretive position. The validity of an appeal to God's ultimate truth is a challenge to the sociologist. The challenge of truth is very well described by Richard Holloway (2001). Selwyn Hughes's (2001) daily readings are based on the assumption that the Bible offers us ultimate and non-negotiable truth. His work is a very good example of this position.

One of the specific areas of enquiry was how the chaplains identified spiritual need. The extract below is taken from the final report and shows how chaplains and patients distinguish between religious and spiritual need.

Box 11.2. Extract from report

Religious and spiritual care needs

Chaplaincy is characterised by both spiritual and religious care giving. The balance of these care-giving activities has shifted over the years for the reasons outlined earlier in this report. It is the language of the 'new universal spirituality' which provides the common currency for the professional discourse of chaplaincy. The changes and ongoing transitions within chaplaincy that were described by chaplains in both sets of interviews, show the degree to which chaplaincy has taken up this universal spiritual care agenda and how it has become formalised into the professional identity of chaplains.

One respondent noted that:

Chaplaincy has gone through a paradigm shift. The focus is no longer on religious care but on spiritual care. (Int. C5, s. 2.1, p. 9)

However, religion remains significant; but it is now located primarily within the private lives of chaplains rather than within the public practice of chaplaincy. There was also a general feeling that the:

> Christian bit . . . is really important, spirituality is important, but mustn't lose other bit. (Int. C34, s. 4, pp. 70–73)

These extracts seem to encapsulate something of the complicated and sometimes confused thinking around the relationship between spiritual care and religious care. There is no doubt that chaplains, and in particular full-time chaplains, are now expected to 'deliver' spiritual care. This is fleshed out by one respondent thus:

> Religious care is meeting people's religious needs, in terms of service and sacraments. Spiritual care, much more person-centred, relates to what makes you tick, feelings, emotions, big questions, meaning. There is a cross over if (you are) Christian. Religious ritual can be empty, sometimes there is more depth to spirituality than religious ritual. (Int. C29, s. 3.10, p. 45)

The comments of this particular chaplain echo the experiences of many people we engaged with:

> spiritual care is acknowledging (that the) person (you are) speaking to is a spiritual person, with spiritual needs, these needs being manifested by first order questions, why is this happening? How am I going to cope? . . . Part of that . . . to understand their search in life, their understanding, what they've made of God, within their own religious context, faith, spiritual aspects goes into that. (Int. C17, s. 5.6, pp. 83–86)

The shift towards spiritual care and away from solely religious care is evident in the way in which the nature of chaplaincy has developed between interview one and two. The guidelines issued in the Health Directive Letter mentioned previously have precipitated a further movement into spiritual care. The requirement to set up spiritual care departments and the possibility of changing the names of the chaplains to 'spiritual care givers' has given a bureaucratic nudge to an increasing trend. This is a very significant departure from the traditional position of chaplain as Christian minister and has raised some dilemmas for chaplains who see themselves first and foremost as Christian ministers. Spiritual ministers tend to have a much wider constituency or at least have a broader remit. Others have said that they like the breadth of the guidelines, their inclusivity and the fact that it is not just a Christian or sacramental agenda, but a wider spiritual care agenda.

The religious care provided by chaplains is characterised by the delivery of formal services such as weddings and funerals, Bible reading, prayer and discussions about God and faith, and sacraments such as baptism and the administration of the Eucharist. However, the delivery of religious care in hospitals is sometimes quite different from the way it is carried out in parish settings. What often occurs is a non-traditional delivery of traditional religious rites and rituals. As Lyall (2001) comments, 'Chaplains will recognise that pastoral practice drives a coach and horse through traditional sacramental theology – or perhaps forces us to reformulate our theology of the sacraments in the light of pastoral practice'.

Religious care is still an integral and important part of chaplaincy, and appears to involve a reasonable amount of a chaplain's time. Some particular groups of people, for instance older people, may be the recipients of more obvious religious care. Religious care may be requested when chaplains are specifically called out. This is particularly so in maternity and children's hospitals when babies may have been stillborn or are seriously ill. There may be something distinct about the chaplain's role as the bearer of religious narratives that despite the spiritual changes in society, people identify with and continue to value.

Chaplains may also facilitate religious care for individuals by contacting their minister, priest, rabbi, imam etc., if the patient wishes. Chaplains may also be seen to have knowledge of, or at least be a starting point for information about, religious issues. An example of this in one of the case studies was a chaplain who was approached by a couple of different staff members about a patient on the ward who was a Jehovah's Witness and asked to facilitate appropriate religious support.

The needs led service culture

The current trend towards needs led services expressed in both health and social care legislation and manifest in Scotland in the patient-centred focus policy, constantly runs up against the difficulties of professional expertise, legal requirements of practice and limited resources. The idea of needs led services is often tempered considerably in practice by the reality of the availability of service, the availability of skill and a realistic knowledge of real needs. Chaplaincy is arguably one of the few roles within the hospital that could truly be needs led. Its declared central concern is to be needs led and patient centred. There may be a tension here with the other central concern, as ministers of the church, to love and to serve God and to enable others to do the same. This task implies the possibility of creating new needs and perhaps challenging expressed needs, rather than simply responding to declared needs. This, once again, raises the question of how far chaplains see themselves as ministers of the church and if they do, what kind of theology underpins their needs led responses?

If chaplaincy sees itself as a profession that has no remit other than to meet spiritual need in a way that is universally meaningful to the needer, must we conclude that spiritual need is anything that the needer says it is? Are there moral boundaries that define acceptable and unacceptable forms of spirituality? If there are, does this mean that spiritual need must be *inter-*

preted by the spiritual care giver, and in effect triaged into different categories?

We have already noted that the chaplains tended to make a distinction between spiritual and religious forms of spirituality. Some saw spiritual need as 'a-religious' in practice. Their work is motivated by their Christian faith but their practice is not necessarily specifically Christian. This raises some important issues relating to what it means for a chaplain to be a health care *professional* in the technical sense of this word. If chaplains perceive themselves to be providing 'spiritual care' which is self-consciously *not* linked to a religious tradition and which downplays the professional significance of ordination, then clearly chaplaincy is a job that can be performed by anyone with expertise in 'spirituality' broadly defined.

It also raises the question as to what specific expertise chaplains are called to offer. Chaplains, like the majority of health care employees, are employed on the basis of their task-specific expertise. The porter is employed to port, the cleaner to clean and the nurse to nurse etc. The extreme specialisation that is prevalent within society in general and hospitals in particular means that tasks and professional expertise are minutely defined as part of the value-for-money trend. Chaplains therefore have to find a specialist area that is identifiable as the specialist area for chaplains. This is potentially in direct contrast to the idea that spiritual need and spiritual care are the province of all. McSherry (2000) raises some interesting and important issues in this area. Denominational religious care is much more easy to specialise in than universal spiritual care. The spiritual care-giving chaplain administers spiritual support to anybody who says they need it in any way that they have defined it. This is an unsatisfactory way to proceed given the set-up of the NHS. It is a challenge for chaplains to both find their niche and to preserve their free floating eye.

The data is able to tell us something of the way in which the chaplains 'find their work', that is, the way they find people with whom to work. It also tells us how the chaplains define the needs of patients. Together, these two sections tell us the core task of chaplaincy. It also tells us something of how spiritual care and religious care are seen as points on a continuum.

What are the needs that patients present to the chaplains?

The data on patient need is drawn from the second set of interviews wherein the question was asked directly, as it had emerged as a significant issue from the 'typical day' data collected in the first set of interviews and from the patient interviews throughout the three case studies ($n = 21$).

In analysing the data it became clear that patients and staff define spiritual need partly in terms of the methods utilised in meeting the need. So, such things as talking and listening are seen as both ways of identifying need, and modes of responding to it.

Availability

Patients assumed that chaplains would speak to anyone and that a major part of their role was to offer comfort, to talk and to encourage people in times of distress and concern.

> She thought that them coming into the wards could encourage other people too – them coming in with cheer. (Inf. Int. P3, 2 December 2003')

Patients tended to make a fairly clear association between chaplains and religion. Some were clear that they did not need to see or want to see a chaplain because they did not consider themselves to be religious. However, they understood and happily accepted that other people might want to see a chaplain.

> He thought that the chaplain provides the same services as he does on the outside, folk who need him, want him, folk really ill, can comfort relatives (think he meant service in the broader sense). He said there were also services that you could attend that were non-denominational. (Int. CP1, 24 November)
>
>   He thought that the chaplain played an essential part for some people. . . . Those of own faith, people needing comfort, people to talk to, essential. People may not be fit enough to go to services. He didn't think the chaplain would be interested if they were an atheist. Said they were 'there to do a job'. Part of this was listening. He thought a lot of people would take heart from this, someone who cares. He said there was a lot of death on this ward, thought chaplains would attend to families. (Int. CP1, paragraph 14)
>
>   She spoke of a minister doing a service for people who may not know who you are or who they are but when there is a service, there is a reaction, something is touching them inside.

Patients' expressed spiritual needs seem to fall into four main categories:

- religious need
- existential need
- teleological need
- practical need.

Sometimes all four categories were expressed at once, or one led naturally into another.

Religious/sacramental needs

These needs were specifically identified as they related to an active, practising faith. Patients wanted to pray, read from scripture, take communion, worship, read the liturgy, and/or have the clergyman/chaplain perform a recognisable religious rite for them or with them. These overtly religiously oriented spiritual needs are perhaps the easiest to identify and meet. It is interesting to note that these services, in a sense, belong to the 'old, religious paradigm' of chaplaincy, which continues to exist alongside the emerging 'spiritual' paradigm. Such a continuation and merging of paradigms is very much in line with the literature which seeks to explore the nature of paradigms and paradigm shifts. It seems that chaplains are experiencing paradigm tension, which is a necessary precursor of paradigm shifts (Kuhn 1970).

Existential need

This expression of need comes out of a situation in which the patients find themselves challenged as to the meaning of their life and/or their illness experience. As people begin to experience themselves differently through the experience of illness ('I'm not feeling myself today'), so they begin to recognise and ask questions which otherwise might not be asked.

The chaplain was there at this time of existential crisis and change, to talk and to ponder together on deep questions of meaning. Patients felt that when in hospital their search for meaning in what was happening became acute. The chaplain's task was to work with the patient to help him or her to find that meaning even if the person is not religious.

Most of the patients interviewed confirmed the dislocation felt on entering hospital and being ill. Being ill requires, as we have already noted, a serious adjustment in the mind of the ill person. This is not always welcome and this adjustment is expressed via a number of different psychological states – anger, sadness, fear and so on.

> He thought that people needed more care after diagnosis and the family too. There's still a psychological/spiritual dimension. He later said that there was more than the psychological dimension, it doesn't give strength or comfort, it gives explanation. (Int. P3, 24 November 2003, Paragraph 12)

The chaplains are thus seen to have an important role as interpreters and translators of experience, who seek to help people explain and understand the answers to their existential questions. The importance of this existential dimension was supported by responses from the chaplains.

> Spiritual needs have a transcendent element, has to have element of existential stuff – who I am, why am I here? – issues of meaning and being, frightening questions that none of us fully examine. Part of our role is to help people find meaning in what is happening. Spirituality is what the person thinks it is. (2nd Int. C36, 4 March 2004, paragraph 180)

Teleological need

By 'teleology' we mean a belief in or the perception of purposeful development toward an end. This idea suggests that there is evidence of purpose of design in the universe and in personal experience. Questions of teleology tend to revolve around some concept of God or transcendent power.

Teleological needs are often expressed by deliberate reference to God's actions and responsibilities in the world in general, and in the particular experience of patients. The very presence of the chaplain (at least when understood as the bearer of a religious narrative) often prompts some form of teleological discussion, partly because both staff and patients assume that that is what the chaplain is there to do. Examples here are questions such as: Why is God punishing me? What have I done to deserve this? Does God love me? However, with the movement towards chaplains as spiritual carers in the more general sense, wherein the religious narratives have less explanatory power, and where understandings of spirituality do not demand transcendence, it may be that this role as teleological guide becomes less significant in the work of the chaplain. Alternatively, the teleological role may change in a way that makes the chaplain a type of 'life-coach', whose primary task is to help patients answer teleological questions without any reference to the supernatural.

Practical need

This refers to issues that worry patients as they move from their normal roles into the role of patient. Here there are practical worries that require some help. These can include looking after children, securing a person's possessions and housing, informing neighbours and family of their current position, getting help to look after pets, financial safety and so forth.

A hierarchy of needs?

The chaplains seem to understand spiritual need as being about exploring the questions surrounding the meaning of life, questions which are triggered by the experience of illness and which confront individuals and families with questions about meaning which are not always comfortable or welcome.

The implication in the data is that the more serious the illness, the more pressing the spiritual need. Mitchell (1999) shows us that there are three types of need which are prioritised by chaplains:

- baby deaths or grave illness;
- cancer deaths – sudden or untimely;
- traumatic emergencies where death or utterly life-changing events are a possibility.

Within the current study these three situations were most commonly discussed and clearly prioritised by the chaplains. While chaplains are clearly sensitive to spiritual needs in general, it appears that these 'loud shouts' for spiritual help are heard most acutely by the chaplains.

An extract from the case study material offers some support to this suggestion:

Chaplains believe that all patients have spiritual needs and that at some time or other many patients will wish to use chaplaincy. Staff saw chaplaincy very much as a service when in need, interventionist, ongoing supportive until the need subsides. Chaplains would like to be in a position to offer more long-standing support to those they had contact with but felt unable to do so because of time commitments. When a patient is distressed, needs a ritual, bereavement, funeral arrangement, needs counselling, or when staff are low, having family problems, or having just experienced a trauma on ward.

Staff recognise the spiritual needs of patients as a dictum they have learned at college, but less than half (staff spoken to) could actually describe gener-alised spiritual needs of individual patients and constantly merged spiritual with religious need, only seeing specific needs such as a patient's need to go to church and to have communion.

Staff indicated that chaplains were there to support staff as well. This was always a reflected support – other folk may need that sort of thing. Spiritual needs were equated with emotional breakdown, bereavement crises. Gener-alised spiritual need, or ongoing spiritual support were not part of the health care workers' vocabulary either for themselves or for their patients. They tended to see spiritual care as a form of intervention in crises. Chaplains also described their spiritual care services in these terms. (s. 2, p. 21)

CONCLUDING REMARKS

HOW DO WE KNOW THAT THIS IS THE CORRECT INTERPRETATION OF WHAT THE CHAPLAINS SAID?

Applying the justice maxim of innocent until proved guilty is quite helpful here. The short answer is that we cannot know if we have provided a correct interpretation but we can become more confident as we publish and present our interpretations and find that they are agreed with both intuitively and in terms of the other studies and literature available. If the chaplains are saying that our interpretations sound about right then, until someone comes up with alternative, better interpretations, ours remain reasonably helpful and accu-rate. We have called this *resonance* elsewhere (Swinton & Mowat 2005). What we must be able to say is that we have used the data available to us, collected in good faith and with an internal rigour, to formulate our interpretations. We assume, for instance, that our participants and respondents did not set out to deceive us and that the researchers did their best to record what they under-stood to be the 'situation'.

As can be seen, we have used an interpretive style of reporting. The style of the report has been to give our interpretations of the data from the beginning of the section rather than to offer 'findings' separate from interpretation. This report was largely written by the two grant holders with first-draft contribu-tions from the researchers involved, who had by that time moved on to other projects/jobs. The grant holders had access to the data rather than the researchers at this stage. This presents a logistical problem of large qualitative data sets being held in one place.

The conclusions and recommendations attempt to rework the interpretations into something practical and useful. We supported our interpretations, our analysis, by referring to other studies, to literature and to the data. We also attempted to triangulate (Denzin & Lincoln 1998) the interpretive work. There were a number of features of this kind of 'triangulation'.

There was member checking acknowledged widely as part of a trustworthy method. This meant returning to the chaplains in the second interviews to check out hunches derived from the first interviews, but also sending the executive summary of the final report to all the chaplains prior to finalising the draft. It also involved asking two theologians to read the final report, as well as a lead training chaplain. Their comments were incorporated into the final text. The two researchers were specifically asked to comment about the ethnographic material, which they did.

This interpretive style allows us to move from 'findings', which have a static and finite quality, to commentary, which is more of a process. Thus we opted for a process account of our findings. This is quite familiar in sociology and theology but not in the more scientific communities. These communities have a fairly unbending structure by which research is reported, and the blending of findings with interpretation proves challenging for readers with this particular vision of research.

CLOSING REMARKS

HOW USEFUL IS THIS REPORT?

Can we say anything universal within the report? The aim of the report was to capture the role of the Scottish hospital chaplain. However, it also, as seen, sought to think about the nature of spiritual need in order that the work of the chaplains could be better understood.

Is the fact that we cannot say anything conclusive and ultimately truthful in the report a failure of method or a fact of interpretation? One way to tackle this question is to consider what other methods might have been used to answer the question *What do chaplains do?* We could have counted the number of ward visits, conducted a time and motion study with chaplains. We could have established the number of minutes used to speak with patients, we could have noted the number of patients on different wards who spoke to or used chaplaincy services. We could have counted the tasks performed by the chaplains and produced a chart of most favoured tasks to least conducted tasks.

This, however, would not have told us anything of chaplaincy in motion and would not have taken into account the enormous variation in personality across the chaplain group, the power of personality to shape actions, the change in actions depending on extraneous circumstances and internal feelings and so on.

These dilemmas leave us wondering how useful the report will be. This will depend largely on the way it is read. It will also depend on the after-sales service provided by the grant holders. By this I mean the presentations and workshops offered that can explore the value of the report. This requires a strong constitution and a fairly open diary. This kind of 'sales' work may be anathema to the purist researcher but is part of the modern-day research task and should be considered at the research proposal stage.

REFERENCES

Austin. J. A. (1998) Why patients use alternative medicine: results of a national study. *Journal of the American Medical Association* **279**(19), 1548–1553.

Browning, D. S. (1983) *Practical Theology*. Harper & Row, San Francisco, CA.

Cobb, M., Robshaw, V. (1998) *The Spiritual Challenge of Health Care*. Churchill Livingstone, Edinburgh.

Coffey, A. (1999) *The Ethnographic Self*. Sage, Thousand Oaks, CA.

Davie, G. (1994) *Religion in Britain since 1945: Believing without Belonging*. Blackwell, Oxford.

Denzin, N. K., Lincoln, Y. S. (1998) *Collecting and Interpreting Qualitative Materials*. Sage, Thousand Oaks, CA.

Denzin, N. K., Lincoln, Y. (2000) *Handbook of Qualitative Research*, 2nd edn. Sage, T Publications Inc., London and California.

Dowie, A. (2002) *Interpreting Culture in a Scottish Congregation*. Peter Lang, New York.

Fry, P. S. (2000) Religious involvement, spirituality and personal meaning for life: existential predictors of psychological wellbeing in community-residing and institutional care elders. *Aging and Mental Health* **4**, 375–387.

Goodall, H. L. (2000) *Writing the New Ethnography*. AltaMira, Lanham, MD.

Hay, D. (1990) Religious Experience Today: Studying the Facts. Cassell, London.

Heelas, P., Woodhead, L., Seel, B., Tusting, K., Szerszynoki, B. (2005) *The Spiritual Revolution. Why Religion is Giving Way to Spirituality*. Blackwell, Oxford.

Holloway, R. (2001) *Doubts and Loves: What is Left of Christianity*. Canongate Books, Edinburgh.

Hughes, S. (2001) *Getting the Best from the Bible*. CWR, Farnham.

Iler, W., Obershain, D., Camac, M. (2001) The impact of daily visits from chaplains on patients with chronic obstructive pulmonary disease COPD: a pilot study. *Chaplaincy Today* **17**, 5–11.

Koenig, H., McCullough, M., Larson, D. (2001) *Handbook of Religion and Health*. Oxford University Press, Oxford.

Kuhn, T. S. (1970) *The Structure of Scientific Revolutions*, 2nd enlarged edn. University of Chicago Press, Chicago, IL.

Larson, D. B., Swyers, J. P., McCullough, M. (1997) *Scientific Research on Spirituality and Health: A Consensus Report*. National Institute for Healthcare Research, Rockville, MD.

Lyall, D. (2001) Spiritual institutions. In H. Orchard (ed.) *Spirituality in Health Care Contexts*. Jessica Kingsley, London.

McLeod, J. (2001) *Qualitative Research in Counselling and Psychotherapy* (p. 3). Sage, London.

McSherry, W. (2000) Education issues surrounding the teaching of spirituality. *Nursing Standard* **14**(42), 40–43.

Mitchell, D. (1999) How do whole time health care chaplains in Scotland understand and practice spiritual care? *Scottish Journal of Healthcare Chaplaincy* **2**(2).

Mowat, H., Swinton, J. (2005) What do chaplains do? The role of the chaplain in meeting the spiritual needs of patients. Report no. CSHD/MR001, February, Mowat Research Ltd, Aberdeen (ISBN 0-9549901-0-2).

Murray, S. A., Kendall, M., Boyd, K., Worth, A., Benton, T. F. (2004) Exploring the spiritual needs of people dying of lung cancer or heart failure: a prospective qualitative interview study of patients and their carers. *Palliative Medicine* **18**, 39–45.

Orchard, H. (2000) *Hospital Chaplaincy: Modern, Dependable?* Sheffield Academic Press, Sheffield.

Robson, C. (2002) *Real World Research*. Blackwell, Oxford.

Scottish Executive (2001) *Cancer in Scotland: Action for Change*. Scottish Executive, Edinburgh.

Scottish Executive (2002) *Spiritual Care in NHS Scotland*. Health Department Letter 76. Scottish Executive, Edinburgh.

Scottish Executive (2003) *A New Public Involvement Structure for NHS Scotland*. Scottish Executive, Edinburgh. Available at: www.scotland.gov.uk/Publications/2003/03/16552/19088. Accessed January 2006.

Smith, B. (1990) In R. J. Hunter (ed.) Dictionary of Pastoral Care and Counselling (p. 136). Abingdon Press, Nashville, TN.

Swinton, J., Mowat, H. (2005) *Practical Theology and Qualitative Research Methods*. SCM, London.

Woodward, J. (1998) A study of the role of the acute health care chaplain in England, PhD thesis, Open University, Milton Keynes.

12 Using Narrative in Care and Research: The Patient's Journey

JOHN ATKINSON

School of Health Nursing and Midwifery, University of Paisley, UK

INTRODUCTION

This chapter will describe and reflect on the development of recording individuals' experience, in a research context, as a method of improving health and social care. As has been seen in other chapters, particularly social anthropology, qualitative methodologies have been eliciting insight and meaning from the observation of human behaviour for many generations. What is less well advanced is how to combine results and analysis gained from, for example, biological science, into a cohesive care 'package' taken up by sufficient numbers of a population.

To this end health care researchers and others have developed a 'bilingual' approach to research activity, using quantitative and qualitative methodologies; for example, establishing a rigorous demographic, statistical and biometric context from a sample cohort combined with an examination of the individuals' experience. I have carried out a number of these studies, in particular a study of nursing intervention with homeless men (Atkinson 2000).

An important part of these and other studies is the use of narrative or stories, often describing the individual's 'journey' or specific experience during a set of events, such as an illness and course of treatment. Whereas, in a common-sense way, the reader or policy maker may see how useful this approach may be, it must also be considered how fragile this source of knowledge is. Do we really expect decisions to be made and large amounts of public money spent on the evidence of a few stories?

This chapter will attempt to face this 'devil' in the eye, exploring the challenges and outlining possible pathways to resolution and incorporation. The chapter also reflects the many discussions held with students and colleagues from the spectrum of research endeavour, and is therefore not presented as a densely argued thesis. I hope that this chapter will combine some of the themes

Interdisciplinary Research: Diverse Approaches in Science, Technology, Health and Society.
Edited by J. Atkinson and M. Crowe.
Copyright © 2006 by John Wiley & Sons, Ltd.

from previous chapters to promote a positive and changed outlook on the future of readers' research practice and interdisciplinary activity.

ETHICS AND RESEARCH GOVERNANCE

Any research involving people – human subjects – is subject to ethical approval and strict research governance and scrutiny. This chapter will not explore these important overarching drivers. However, the guiding biomedical philosophical and ethical principles of autonomy, justice, beneficence and non-malfeasance underpin all research that seeks to gain the individual's experience.

Specifically in relationship to health and social care there is recognition of tension between the personal autonomy of the individual, his or her needs, the state or providers' capacity or willingness to provide them and the professions' opinion of how important they are. Also, whereas there may be a general underpinning of *social justice*, evidence-based care which is value for money is driven by precepts of *distributive justice* and the utilitarian principle of the greatest good for the greatest number.

Distributive justice also impinges on beneficence, the doing of good for patient or population. Any effort spent on 'good' action must be accountable in terms of its proven effect on the target – just generally 'making things better' is often insufficient. Similarly, in a more litigious environment when any action can have unexpected consequences, non-malfeasance is not confined to officials or formal carers doing bad things to patients or clients. Defensive practice examines the risk of the potentially good action causing unforeseen harm. Thus one may discover a person or population's need and its remedy but one still has to find other people to take the risk and enact the solution. Qualitative, story-gathering research can be a useful tool in this dilemma

WHY STORIES SHOULD NOT BE USED IN RESEARCH

STORIES ARE NOT TRUE

There is a wonderfully moving story, originally a novella, subsequently turned into a beautiful animated film by Frederic Back, called 'The Man who Planted Trees' by Jean Giono. I sometimes give the book or show the video to students. It tells the story of a young Frenchman returning from the horrors of World War One. He decides to take a walking holiday in the Haute Provence. He meets a shepherd and his dog. The shepherd lives entirely alone and does not speak much. Every day he plants 100 or so acorns and other tree seeds or saplings.

Over the next 40 years the young man returns to visit the shepherd, who continues his task against the odds of weather and vermin. Gradually the land comes to life. Rivers return, people begin to live there and forests emerge as it used to be in Roman times. So gradual is this progress and on such a large scale that everyone thinks that the regeneration is a miracle or freak natural phenomenon. The shepherd, Elezeard Bouffier, grows old and dies in a shelter in Banon. The details of his death add authority to the tale. The story conveys great 'truth' – except that it did not happen and it is not true.

In 1953 Giono was asked by Reader's Digest to write a story about an unforgettable character, on the assumption that the character would be real. Giono changed this to the character he *thought* would be the most unforgettable! He also gave the copyright of the story to the world. The story has much to convey if one prefaces the text with: 'If someone was to undertake this activity over 40 years, these would be some likely results . . .'. It also has 'truth' in that it encourages the research student, for example, to take a steady and methodical approach. It would be difficult to transfer the story further than this – that is, from the general 'truths' or insights.

STORIES ARE TRUE

In the political field, stories or vignettes are often used to exemplify the shortcomings of opponents' policies. Even though these stories are based on actual events, they are often soon discredited. Errors in factual detail are highlighted, but often more damaging, differences of interpretation are made. In 1992 in the UK General Election the 'War of Jennifer's Ear' was a famous case itself named after an eighteenth-century conflict. So, even when stories are true they can be unreliable or dangerous.

In terms of research, the carefully captured vignette can also be vulnerable. Does the research study carried out in the remote and rural setting of South West Scotland (Atkinson et al. 2002) have any relevance to the inner city study (McPherson & Leydon 2001)? On first consideration the answer may be, probably not, especially if one tries to consider 'like with like'. As will be seen later, comparisons were made in these two studies but they had to be precisely described.

STORIES ARE MANIPULATIVE

Individual stories are often profoundly moving and reach across cultural and other divides. As listeners and readers, we engage with sadness and tragedy, often imagining ourselves in a similar situation. How much should this be taken into account?

On a BBC Radio 4 programme (*File on Four*, November 2005) the process of getting new prescription drugs appraised, onto the market and into patients was described. Differences were highlighted between the length of time appraisals took between Scotland and the rest of the UK. The 'story' of this process was juxtaposed with the stories of individuals, presently suffering with cancer or other life threatening disease. The clash of these two perspectives was dramatic – the plodding uncaring bureaucracy versus the desperate individual. However, one could imagine the counter-story if 'life saving' drugs were rushed onto the market with corresponding mistakes. Even when a balanced approach is taken, as can be witnessed in this programme, it may be difficult to see how this approach assists the policy makers or the individual patients.

Phrases often used in this context are 'Creating heat but no light' and 'Sad cases make bad laws'. The stories are seen to detract from objectivity and focusing on the 'real' issues.

STORIES ARE DISTRACTING

The problem of manipulation is sometimes compounded by the problem of stories distracting from the 'main issue'. If one takes the issue of the campaigns to get immunisation uptake increased in the population, for example, the measles, mumps and rubella (MMR) vaccine, usually given together as a triple dose, the 'main issue', surely, is that it is vital to get an over 90% uptake of the vaccine. This level of immunisation provides what is termed 'herd immunity'; any less than this level creates a real danger that these diseases will break out in the community. The compromise position of giving the three vaccines as single doses over time heightens the chances of non-compliance and leaves the community vulnerable.

The 'case' put in this way is objective and true. It would be difficult to argue against it and scientific evidence will support it. Surely all of us engaged in health care must put all other distractions aside to 'get over' this message?

And yet, as the father of a child with a severe disability, who was diagnosed at the age when widely published stories warned about the possible dangers of the 'triple' vaccine, how am I to respond? My personal experience, and that of many others, of measles, mumps and rubella was not dramatic. Many people have never experienced them and know very few people who have. Those that have first- or second-hand experience may look at the balance of risk of contracting a childhood infection, which most people appear to survive, and the possibility of looking after a severely disabled child for life.

My wife's and my personal experience of parenting a disabled child – with its concomitant impact on life, relationships, earning capacity on the, usually female, main carer in a world that demands two earners – has been augmented and supported by undertaking a study examining the needs of severely disabled children (Atkinson & Kennedy 2002). Many people in the community have second-hand experience of witnessing a family like ours. They may be basing their decision not to vaccinate on what they have seen (and what they say they know) and what they have not.

In another public health campaign a few years ago, there was a drive to reduce hypothermia among the elderly. The campaign concentrated on the scientifically correct activities to 'Keep the heat IN'. One of the challenges raised in the evaluation was that many people in the target group did not recognise or relate to the idea of keeping heat in. However, they did have knowledge and experience of the scientifically incorrect 'Keeping the cold OUT'. Apparently only heat exists, cold is the absence of heat.

Given the *true* facts, how can we research and intervene with people whose perceptions are often untrue? Is it just a question of hammering home the 'science'? Or are bridges and accommodation made?

In the case of health care service delivery there is growing recognition that pragmatism and uneasy alliances have to be enacted. This does not change the essential truth of the science, but recognises that if one wants to put it into practice other factors are involved.

PERCEPTIONS, SCIENCE, METHODOLOGY AND HEALTH CARE

In other fields too, there is similar recognition. While preparing this book I have discussed with its authors, particularly those from traditional scientific backgrounds, these 'distracting' factors. Andrew Hursthouse, the geo-environmentalist, pointed out that endeavour on land, such as the central belt of Scotland, which has been industrially worked and polluted for 200 years, is different from operating in virgin rain forest. This difference impacts on the science. Similarly, Ian Boyd, the marine biologist, described how pods of whales are 'owned' by different indigenous people in different parts of the whales' migratory journey. People's perception and response to their environment influences the science.

Returning to health and social care, the bridges and accommodation of competing factors may be considered as follows: a rough, though not strict, continuum between quantitative and qualitative enquiry is created, each facet supporting the whole.

STRUCTURE, FUNCTION AND PROCESS

At the quantitative end of enquiry one tracks by empirical observation the classic pathways of Cartesian causal links – infectious diseases being one of the first historical examples of tracing the relationship between specific micro-organisms, populations, individuals and named diseases. The interaction between structure (arrangement of parts), function (procedural role) and process (how the result is achieved) is established. Much of this endeavour may happen at a distance, in a laboratory, for example. However, even today the fieldwork at the site is important.

Today microbiology is seen as one of the 'harder' sciences, where narrative would have very little place. This would be mistaken. As has been seen in

Chapter 1 and running throughout the book, there is the need to establish a hypothesis – or 'likely story' – to begin the enquiry. One of the greatest likely stories generated the massive Victorian development of the London sewers by Joseph Bazalgette. The need to pump water and sewage away from the city was based on the story and belief that the smell carried disease. This was subsequently found to be flawed; nevertheless, it did impact on the real cause, micro-organisms.

Part of the solution came from the careful observation and story collection of Dr John Snow after the 1855 cholera outbreak in Broad Street, London (the original account may be found at www.ph.ucla.edu/epi/snow/snowbook_a2.html). Tracing the use of the water pump, he found that the brewery workers did not suffer from cholera as they only drank beer, whereas a woman who had bottles from the pump and who lived some distance away died. Epidemiology combines the microbiological enquiry with the population-based observation.

Today we hear similar likely stories from astrophysics as we try to make sense of the structure, function and process of the universe. As in 1855, it sometimes appears that what we are asked to believe by scientists is much more outlandish than anything from religion! Over time the stories are refined, adapted or rejected and renewed.

Adaptation in care research concentrates on function and process. Once a scientific or policy principle is established, it then has to be activated generally. The inter-relationship between the original principle and how it is enacted often changes, even if the original principle remains the same. New technology or techniques become available or fresh knowledge overtakes. As a nurse, over 30 years I have witnessed how procedures that used to be highly specialist, requiring considerable human intervention and expertise, are now mechanically operated. This change is noteworthy not only in terms of quantitative observation and audit, it also forms the basis of other enquiry.

CONTENT, MEANING AND VALUE

Having established the objective, quantitative evidence, process – how people do things – often also forms the beginning of qualitative enquiry, in particular if it is combined as 'how and why?'. If formal care is seen as the institutional response to scientific knowledge and government policy, demanding considerable public funding, then a volatile mix of knowledge, belief and political conviction ensues, which sometimes requires unpicking to enable progress.

The emphasis of enquiry shifts from proof to insight, prediction to perspective. What is the content (substantive or meaningful parts), meaning and value to the participants of this situation? What does the present practice or procedure represent to the participants apart from its primary function? Insight gained from these and similar lines of enquiry can assist in the implementation of more objective evidence.

UNIVERSALITY, UTILITY, VALUE FOR MONEY

Health and social care research is pragmatic and seeks solutions. It is anchored by the principles of universality (sometimes called generalisability), utility (it must be useful) and value for money (it is generally resourced from public funds, particularly in the UK). Whereas these may be agreed as good general principles, basing action in reality, from a research perspective it can be problematic, in particular the burden on researchers to predict that their endeavours will coincide with the principles in advance. Whether laboratory experiments or patient care centred studies, one has to use the literature, received wisdom and possibly old stories to predict a contribution to new knowledge. When one considers how many benefits to mankind have happened accidentally or as a by-product of non-associated activity – technology from space exploration, for example – it may be seen that this may influence the type of research in which one engages.

This is not an attack on the principles of usefulness and value for money. However, it is part of the challenge in health and social care to combine the validation of received and known wisdom with radical new thought and change the way we think – the paradigm shift.

PARADIGM SHIFTING: THE IRONBRIDGE STORY

USING THE RECEIVED WISDOM: OLD LIES AND NARROW PATHS

One flaw with using the literature review and received wisdom as a basis for new research is the assumption that knowledge has progressed across a broad front, picking up most of the facts, or what it is possible to know, along the way. Simon Singh's books *Fermat's Last Theorem* and *The Code Book* encapsulate much of the history of mathematics. What they exemplify is the stepping-stone or piggyback nature of advances in knowledge – that is, using one theorem or proof (in the case of mathematics) to take the present endeavour somewhere else. This may be achieved without total knowledge of why something works. In the history of building, formulas and ratios have often been devised centuries before their explanation. These reliable pathways can be narrow, so that twenty-first-century techniques have some limited and fixed features that dictate the outcome.

QUALITATIVE INSIGHT

An example of these knowledge pathways was demonstrated in a BBC2 programme examining how the first iron bridge in the world was built across the River Severn at Ironbridge in 1779 (see www.bbc.co.uk/history/

society_culture/industrialisation/iron_bridge_01.shtml). The essential mystery is that the bridge was constructed in huge pieces, much larger than those used today and in a time when heavy lifting tools were very limited. For many years engineers have tried to discern how it was achieved. Modern methods tend to use platforms and large amounts of supportive trappings and yet there was no evidence of the purchase of the required amount of lumber necessary for this methodology. Among the BBC team were an engineer and an art historian. The latter sought to discover pictures of the bridge under construction, as there were no written accounts.

The historian presented an impressionistic watercolour by the Swedish artist Elias Martin of the iron bridge under construction. The painting (one may call it qualitative evidence) shows the antithesis to what may have been expected using a modern model. Instead of a huge platform and supportive structure, there are two wooden jibs lashed together, looking like rugby (or American football) posts – rather sleek and spindly. In 2001 the team, with the help of the Royal Engineers, built a half-sized model to test this surprising methodology. It worked.

What has also been interesting has been the continued debate since the experiment. Just because the experiment worked does not, of course, mean that that was how it was done. However, it does present insight into other ways of achieving a result, a paradigm shift.

Health and social care research benefits from a combination of quantitative and qualitative approaches. This is sometimes called 'bilingual' research. The rest of this chapter will describe aspects of this work, in particular the collection of stories, describing people's journeys, using exemplars from various projects. The common theme from all the projects has been the discovery and description of paradigm shifts.

EXEMPLARS: OVERARCHING THEMES

EVIDENCE BASE: GOAL AND CURSE

This part of the chapter will use four exemplars of health care projects to demonstrate the use of stories, vignettes or paradigms to elucidate important themes. Perhaps the most important overarching theme is that stories can help present solutions to ameliorate the impact of evidence-based care on the individual. The drive of evidence is to cure in the most useful, generalisable and value for money way possible. This precept is similar to the travel industry – which should perhaps be termed the 'destination' industry. What the individual feels or experiences is often not as important as the end result. One endures discomfort today for putative benefit tomorrow. The procedures, rituals and services of yesteryear to ensure individual comfort, for example, are sometimes sacrificed to the principles of cure. This is not a criticism; however, what is interesting is that often the comfort or feelings of the individual do affect the final result. One can also discover that although human presence or interaction may not have a positive primary effect (e.g. cure), they have a beneficial supportive role.

In the 1987 King's Cross Underground fire in London, which killed 31 people, it was observed that increased automation had lessened the number of staff on duty (Fennell 1988). This had led to a heightened risk as each individual (whatever their primary job) had an important, but formally unrecognised, safety function interacting with and guiding the public – a role sorely lacking in the incident.

In terms of health and social care interventions, treatment and referral are commonly recognised. Assessment and recording (the initial story gathering) are often not seen as intervention. What my own and others' work has shown is that this activity provides the whole basis of care, giving individuals a bureaucratic existence. Also recommending an individual's story to another, advocacy, can have dramatic impact on the group and individual's progress and journey.

The lack of context and story can also have a confusing impact on individuals. A personal experience drove this home while sitting with my father when he was in hospital. As a chef, his whole life was centred on building events and stories in which people journeyed through the important milestones of their lives. As I sat with him one afternoon after he had undergone major surgery, I was amazed at how much excellent evidence-based care he was receiving. Scans, tests and procedures, many of which had previously needed days of waiting and rare specialists, were all focused on him. He appreciated the need for it but he found the complete lack of routine very confusing, like being in an airport lounge just waiting for things to happen. We both reminisced about the 'old' days when each day a drama of routine and ritual was enacted, everyone knowing their place and what they were supposed to do, doctor, nurse and patient, chef and customer.

EXEMPLAR ONE: NURSING HOMELESS MEN

Themes: Using Demography and Stories; Groups and Individuals; Challenging Assumptions

This study (Atkinson 2000) presented health profiles of hostel residents, made assessments, immediate interventions and referrals, evaluated their effect and discovered insights into the residents' experiences. The objectives were addressed by gathering and analysing quantitative and qualitative data. Two hostels were used. The information was gathered by a project nurse, who acted as a practitioner in addition to collecting data for the study. Statistical and qualitative data were collected. This exemplar concentrates on the 'stories' gained from the statistical data.

SUMMARY OF IMPORTANT FINDINGS

Assumption of Access to Care

Nearly all the men in both hostels were found to be registered with a general practitioner and most had seen their doctor within the last 5 months. This information established that, in theory, the men should be able to access services such as community nursing in exactly the same way as the rest of the population. At the time of the study there was no specialist District Nursing or Health Visitor provision; a Community Psychiatric Nursing service had just started. As will be seen in the findings below, this apparently 'normal' ability to access services was influenced by a number of complicating factors. Homeless people do experience difficulty getting care and need assistance from generic and specialist nurses.

The majority of both groups of men attended their doctor regularly. However, they tended to attend mainly to collect sickness certificates or similar low interaction activity. In terms of referral to other health and welfare services, these visits were not productive.

Perceptions of Health

The question 'How do you feel?' proved one of the most useful questions in the study. Over half the sample felt well. Significant statistical relationships were found between those men who stated that they felt unwell or ill and hospital admissions, high levels of anxiety and depression, and high use of Accident and Emergency.

The significance of these findings for nursing practice is that when asked 'How do you feel?' the men answered honestly. An assumption is often made that people in difficult, marginalised situations lie to get something out of you. This view was heard during the study. The evidence presents a challenge to this sceptical view.

Preferences for Companionship and Type of Accommodation

Similarly, asking residents 'Where would you like to live?', 'With whom would you like to live?' and 'Where is home?' provided insight into residents' present well-being and aspirations. Two thirds of the men wanted to live in a house; a third of the men wanted to live in hostel accommodation. Although the largest group wanted to live alone, a third wanted to live with their wife and/or family. Personal aspirations had an effect on how they felt at the present, and on their level of contentment with their circumstances.

The Hospital Anxiety and Depression Scale

Anxiety

The Hospital Anxiety and Depression (HAD) Scale (Zigmond & Snaith 1983) had not been used before with homeless men. A number of health professionals were doubtful about the use of the tool with this group, fearing attention seeking. Again, the notion was disproved. Half of the sample fell within normal score range, a third were in the high range.

Depression

Only a third of the main sample scored in the normal range; a third scored highly. The HAD depression tool isolates treatable clinical, biogenic depression. The levels in both hostels were high. This discovery became one of the most important findings of the study. Biogenic depression is considered treatable and yet none of the men discovered with a high score were being treated. The general assumption was that depression emanated from the bad living conditions; a typical comment was 'Well, he would be depressed, living in that terrible place'.

Interventions

During the first 3 weeks of the study almost all of those assessed required intervention. Interventions were described in three categories – treatments, referrals and advocacy. Advocacy was defined as any action taken on behalf of a resident which supported his 'case'.

Evaluation

Twenty-three GPs received referrals from the project nurse. The referrals were thought appropriate and useful. None of the men with high depression scores were treated or referred for further intervention.

Five District Nurses received referrals from the project nurse. All the nurses were interviewed. Three of the residents received specific nursing interventions, with one taken onto a District Nurse's caseload for continuing monitoring.

The main barrier to the men receiving the full potential of service delivery was seen by the doctors and nurses in universally bleak terms. They did not expect to achieve much with this transient and 'unreliable' group. Action tended to be minimal, concentrating on the main presenting signs. An expert panel of District Nurses, presented with six anonymised cases and asked for care plans, described a potentially more holistic, multidisciplinary 'package'.

Roles Identified in the Study

Proactive Casefinder

In this role (demonstrated by the project nurse) the community nurse acts as a 'generalist' able to make initial assessments of individuals, followed by treatments, referral or advocacy. The nurse can also undertake ongoing monitoring. The project nurse demonstrated a variety of skills and interactions. He was able to identify both physical and psychiatric illness for ongoing referral. Because of the workload and referral patterns under which generic district nurses worked, the role of casefinder as a formal part of their 'core business' was difficult.

Reactive Specialist

In this role and in response to a referral the community nurse performs specific actions, such as ulcer management or instigation of continuing care. The District Nurses who received referrals from the project nurse were seen to act in a reactive specialist role. The monitoring of a population of vulnerable or marginalised people would be ineffective if District Nurses acted only from referrals. In another study of the effectiveness of the referral system as a means of identifying needs for District Nursing, Worth et al. (1995) state:

> There is little evidence of a proactive approach to the identification of need by district nurses at either individual or community level. Potential service users are discouraged from having direct access to district nursing advice and care, the GP acting as the primary gatekeeper. (p. xiii)

As a model for monitoring this and other groups, the project nurse's approach would be more effective as it is more wide ranging. Coordinated hostel population monitoring requires to be planned strategically at a management level, rather than leaving it to individual nurses.

The reactive approach also demonstrated evidence of hostels being treated differently by nurses. One nurse stated that 'her' GP did not like 'his' District Nurses going into the hostels. This pattern of relying on others to filter contact with the hostels and wider community was not universal but was strongly discernible. All the nurses were alert to a possible threat of violence, although there was no actual evidence of nurses being in any more danger in a hostel than in a normal city street. Experienced nurses managed this situation, seeing it as a normal function of their work.

All the District Nurses had heavy workloads as 'reactive specialists'. Time and resources need to be managed systematically to cater for the needs of the homeless and other marginalised people. Merely expecting nurses to 'squeeze' these activities into a busy day is unreasonable and inappropriate.

Discussion

In terms of nursing practice and research influencing policy the combination of statistical and qualitative evidence was seen to be useful when presenting the findings to groups of civil servants, managers and clinicians. The combination of presenting statistical results – describing the groups – followed by the personal story of one or a few individuals to exemplify the case provides extremely powerful evidence at every management level.

Half of the interventions were carried out in the first three weeks and most residents were attending their GPs on a regular basis. Policy makers need to assist health carers to formalise these visits and monitor the health of these and other groups. Specialist nurses may carry out initial assessments. However, generic community nurses are in a useful position to carry out ongoing monitoring. They can, with management support, also develop a special interest in the care of these individuals. From a management perspective designating specific hostels and sites to individual health centres helps to focus intervention and impact.

In regard to everyday practice, therefore, time is not the 'enemy'. Professionals do not need time-consuming studies before making an impact. The important feature of the process was consistent, regular short bursts of attendance. The sessions were more concentrated at the beginning but in a real-life situation this would soon 'level out' to a monitoring role.

A large group of men were found with biogenic depression. Many of these men could have been treated, their depression causal to their homeless state, rather than, as was the professional assumption, that they were depressed as an environmental response. If individuals suffering from depression were treated systematically, then a number may be able to move on and lead more fulfilling lives. At street level it is unhelpful to the individual to assume that mental illness is caused by their homeless state, and is therefore not worth addressing. This can trap the person into a hopeless cycle. All psychological morbidity should be considered worthy of intervention.

Conclusion

No claim is made that this work stands alone in influencing policy. Presentations and assistance to other projects have been enacted at every management and practice level. Along with other health and welfare colleagues, improvements to specialist and generic services have been made. Working with homeless people is not seen as so 'far out' as it was in 1984 (when I first started this work), when access to hostels was often denied. However, there is still much work to be done. This study has, at least, demonstrated that even difficult areas can be systematically examined. Importantly, it also demonstrated that simple questions such as 'How do you feel?' remain an essential tool in the nurse's and researcher's repertoire.

EXEMPLAR TWO: PATIENTS' CANCER JOURNEYS

Themes: Describing Conflicting Experience; Discovering Unknowns; Comparing Remote and Rural with Urban Stories

This exemplar concentrates on the collection of qualitative evidence and actual stories of individuals' experience. Some key methodological issues are also discussed.

The Kintyre area of Argyll in Scotland is a short flight from Glasgow but 4 hours by road. Patients and their carers face challenges when gaining access to cancer care services. As part of a government-funded project, examining current services for patients with cancer, an independent qualitative study was commissioned. The method comprised selecting 30 individuals who had received cancer services within the past 3 years. Using semi-structured interviews, critical incident techniques and prompts, the researcher recorded patients' stories. Two main forms of information were discovered. First, insight was gained into practical issues. These included how airport, health and other services operated. Second, the study discovered the importance of other factors in patients' lives while they were undergoing treatment; for example, patients' experience if they had relatives living near the Glasgow treatment centres. The simple methods used in this study are generalisable in several settings, particularly in communities where local factors may influence the experience of people receiving services from providers situated in a geo-graphically distant location. Perhaps the most important feature, agreed by all parties, was that the insights gained from this study may not have been gained using more 'mainstream' quantitative methods.

Rationale for a Qualitative Approach

Quantitative, statistical analysis is not always desirable when describing more complex experiences as it may hide an individual's experience, as the emphasis is placed on frequency of phenomena and their representative nature. Qualitative analysis recognises events because they are thought important enough to report. Also, the cumulative effect of events is often greater than the sum of its parts, the 'gestalt' effect, described by, among others, Patricia Benner. The study has taken some of her techniques of recording (Benner 1984). In relation to patients suffering pain, Carr (1999) highlights how qualitative methodologies have often been ignored:

> yet they offer understanding and perceptions people have of their own world and how this affects their action. (p. 199)

Data Collection: Critical Incident Recording

The study used the taking of contemporaneous notes and critical incident technique, particularly in relation to the collection of significant events and their analysis (Burnard 1991; Flanagan 1954; Patton 1990). The system is simple at the point of entry and enables collation and analysis at a later date. This study did not use critical incident technique to establish high and low standards (Norman et al. 1992). It used the method of collating data into themes. Norman and Parker (1990) used this technique in an investigation with psychiatric patients encountering hostel life. The technique is achieved by the use of comments, themes and paradigms.

Comments are short sentences or phrases recorded in a diary or on the interview sheet. Comments form the basis for *themes*. The collection and collation of comments enables the researcher to identify certain themes that give insight into the experience of the sample patients. The technique has similarities to grounded theory in that the researcher absorbs the data from the subject without the 'lens' of an external theory. Grounded theory, however, tends to take a broader base of data and by analysis explain phenomena, developing new theory generalisable to other situations (Strauss & Corbin 1998, pp. 275–280). This study used a more focused approach, concentrating on the patient's particular 'cancer' experience (no reference was made to differing living conditions or other social factors, for example). The primary focus is to witness and record the patient's side of the story; no generalisable theory is mooted, although it is hoped that readers experience insight. To ensure that the findings represent a true record, the participating patients had full access to the final report.

Paradigms are stories that describe a situation better than the description of its constituent parts and are also used to exemplify themes. The main aim of the paradigm is to present a story that has created a change of the researcher's perception (a paradigm shift) or knowledge.

In practical terms, the researcher (principal author) kept a contemporaneous diary (a lined cash book, enabling coding) in which he recorded comments and paradigms. He also made margin notes on the patients' forms during interview. The technique is simple and concise, requiring minimal equipment and documentation. This proved to be beneficial when working in remote country areas in bad weather.

Campbeltown Interventions

A few patients had received treatment in Campbeltown, the main town in Kintyre. Many patients liked the idea of receiving treatment nearer home. Strong themes emerged regarding home or local treatment:

> Chemotherapy at home can be 'frightening', particularly if the treatment doesn't go to plan.

Patients described how there was no 'back-up' if something unusual happened:

> Patients perceived that very few treatments were 'off the shelf'.

Patients described how alterations had to be made to their treatment because of their condition and/or following the results of investigations.

Lay Terms

The use of lay terms for treatment was often confusing, unless the health worker ensured the 'message' was precise. One patient blamed him/herself for not getting the right treatment after a very painful experience with one type of bladder washout:

> I'd had this washout thing before and it was very sore, I couldnae walk after it. Sometime after this consultant says 'Well, we'll give you this treatment which is just like a wee washout' and I said 'No way, it's too sore'. So he didn't give it me. Then I found out that it wasn't the sore one but another one. I felt bad because I'd mouthed off and hadn't got the right treatment.

Connected with this theme was a tendency of some health workers to describe the impact of the treatment on the cancer not on the patient's ability to function. One patient graphically put it:

> The nurse was ever so good. She told me how the treatment would attack the cancer in great detail, but she didn't tell me whether I would wet myself on the way home.

Another theme was the heavy impact of check-up appointments and procedures:

> We took four and a half hours to get there on that day, in that silly bus, so we were all a bit stiff. I was sitting waiting to go into the doctor [surgical registrar]. I was called in to see him. I noticed the time was 20 minutes to 1. I went in and sat down. He said 'Hello, how are you?' I said 'Fine'. He came over and squeezed my tummy [she made a squeezing motion with her fingers twice] and said 'OK, that's fine'. I came out and looked at the clock. It was 17 minutes to 1. Then it was four hours home again.

Comparison with Other Studies

The diversity of practical, emotional and other responses found in this study is mirrored in other recent studies. In particular, an Irish study describes women's experience of discovering breast lumps. Coping strategies combined practical problem solving alongside emotionally focused responses (O'Mahony 2001). These interlinking factors were certainly demonstrated in the Kintyre study, where worry for other members of their family sometimes made the individual's own cancer appear peripheral. A report on the BBC Radio 4 *Women's Hour* (4 October 2001) programme highlighted a study of inequalities in cancer care. Dr Michel Coleman from the London School of Hygiene and Tropical Medicine described a qualitative study which discovered similar themes to those discovered in Kintyre in deprived cities in the UK. Of particular note was the lack of a cohesive administrative journey or pathway on which the patient could progress. Also significant was the role of individuals who were central 'lynchpins' to their family, and who subjugated or hid their illness for as long as possible (McPherson & Leydon 2001).

EXEMPLAR THREE: CHILDREN WITH HIV – 'WHEN SOMEBODY KNOWS MY NAME'

Themes: Documentation and the Bestowal of Humanity; Stabilising Context; the Essential Partnership

This exemplar (Atkinson 1993) demonstrates the enacting of story gathering in practice. Of note as well is that although medical science procedures had been introduced, there was something lacking which required a combined quantitative and qualitative approach.

In 1990 I was asked by a charity to assess a project in Romania that was caring for 200 HIV-positive children in hospital and other institutions. The project had a Romanian medical director who was being assisted in her work by two consultants from Britain: a virologist and a community paediatrician with HIV expertise. My role was to make a needs assessment, consult with the medical team, and discover prospective patterns of practice that might improve the children's situation. My own background was as a community nurse with expertise in delivering nursing care to marginalised people in deprived circumstances, particularly those with HIV, and the homeless.

I discovered that although some babies and children were terminally ill, most of them were not. The children were receiving adequate medication. Those who were dying seemed to die not from HIV disease, but from preventable malnutrition and dehydration. Details like name, date of birth, weight and continuing observation charts were not accurate, although injections were given regularly. The children were also, mainly, quiet and docile. They were not treated cruelly although they were not treated as individuals. There was little or no use of their names. These children were not orphans, but when they were admitted they commonly became 'lost'. They became orphans by default because the parents could not find them or felt that it was hopeless to look.

Over the next few months we set up a nursing project using a community model whose main purpose was to individualise the children, and to monitor and encourage their nutrition, hydration, developmental milestones, play and other activities. A full-time team of nurse volunteers worked in two of the main institutions. The use of each child's name was central to this model, and the name, age and date of birth (where known) were placed above each child's bed. The names were also put on the children's plastic bibs.

On subsequent visits the change was dramatic. The mortality and morbidity had improved. Each child had his or her own cot and was always called by name. Documentation had improved, so that it was known more exactly how a child was progressing. This meant that children were not slipping into serious and terminal illness, as happened before. Instead of all the children having uniformed cropped hair, the Romanian staff would bring in little ribbons and make other small differences. Instead of docile, still children, the wards took on the demeanour of a minor riot, with each child shouting for attention or to a friend.

Because it was known who each child was, the team began liaison with the parents. An outpatients clinic was started for children outside as well. This helped prevent children from being lost in the system. The most important process in the project, therefore, happened when the children were called by their names. This had the practical purpose of establishing accurate records, enabling continuity of care, and providing building blocks to rehabilitation.

Naming the children appeared to have a profound effect on the Romanian nursing assistants. Because of the enormity of the problems they faced, with death and despair all around, it must have been difficult to relate to a seemingly endless string of sick and dying children. Although Romanians are renowned for their love of children, this terrible, relentless situation tended to make the workers detach themselves from the individual plight of the children.

Once the children had names and a story (of which they, the workers, were a very important part), there appeared to be more hope around the institutions. Attachments between individuals became common. That small act of naming bestowed humanity on each child. Their individuality was recognised; each had a place in history.

The American nursing theorist Patricia Benner has used this exemplar to demonstrate how the objective 'clinical gaze' sometimes removes medical and health practice from its service and spiritual roots. In an article 'Researching the human spirit' (Schwartz 2003), she observes 'recognition practice':

> Benner calls Atkinson's simple act of naming a 'recognition practice.' Nurses in this country have long talked of the need to incorporate such practices into clinical care. They ask: how can we send heart patients or diabetics home with clinical regimens to follow if we don't understand the world in which they live – their caregivers, living conditions, daily schedules? Without that understanding, aren't the clinical solutions doomed to failure?
>
> These are important concerns, of course, that have clear clinical, even ethical links, but are they spiritual as well? Benner believes they are. 'The recognition practices of those nurses [in Romania] – all recognition practices – are spiritual in that we require a response from others to our existence in the world,' says Benner. 'No one is untouched by spirituality.'
>
> That may be so, but Benner confesses that in spite of the increased attention to the concept, 'We have as much problem as we've ever had in linking the life-social world with biomedicine. How we put them back together is the most pressing problem we have, given our aging population and the prevalence of chronic illness.'

EXEMPLAR FOUR: MOVING A CHILDREN'S SERVICE FROM
A HEALTH TO A SOCIAL MODEL

Themes: Describing Common Need; Exploring Ideologies

This exemplar demonstrates how story-gathering techniques can elucidate movement from one way of operation to another and the impact of the journey.

In a South Scotland Health Board the care of children with severe disabilities was, in part, carried out at a hospital. The staffing of this facility comprised a high level of nursing intervention. Following a reappraisal and change of policy, the care of these children was transferred to a children's charity at a new purpose-built facility. The care in the new centre has a more social focus with a decreased but complementary nursing input that is calibrated according to the specific needs and length of stay. The hospital was closed in June 1999.

Over the past 15 years there has been a considerable shift in the UK from institutionalised, medically oriented care towards a more community centred, social approach (Kirk 1998; Nolan et al. 1996). This has led to a complete rearrangement of the structure, function and process of care delivery. What is less clear is the impact of these changes on the content, experience and value of these services (Hall 1996).

Recent literature tends to emphasise a child/patient-centred, progressive model where the patient/client is constantly exposed to new and encouraging stimuli in a moving environment (Callan et al. 1995). However, some of the literature regarding 'respite' highlights the importance of creating stability for the parents/guardians who are having to cope with a long-term, seemingly unchanging situation (Vanleit & Crowe 2000).

Aims and Objectives

The study set out to describe the present provision of care and report on differing models and perceptions of care and possible dynamic tensions and areas of conflict between new resource carers, parent/guardians and senior management.

The introduction of this new resource produced tension since parents were unhappy about the move from hospital to community and set up an action group against the hospital closure. The tripartite partnership was extended to incorporate parents – which was stated to have resulted in ownership of the service by parents and the creation of parents' group meetings.

Interviews with the Parents: Specific Themes

There was a wide variety of experiences and views regarding their children's care, respite arrangements and particularly the transition from hospital to the new resource. There was general consensus, however, on the value and positive experience that the new resource provides. The themes have been exemplified by quotations from the parents.

The Use of Respite Services

Two main themes emerged regarding why parents use respite services. First, some parents were looking after their disabled child and sometimes other children by themselves, that is without a full-time partner. Second, parents with other children often use the respite time to engage in activities with those siblings. Subsidiary to these themes was that some parents wished their children to be 'part of the system' and be used to other people by the time they were of adult age. By adult age, many perceived that their children would require more respite care. Some parents expressed how the respite time also allowed them to undertake other activities, at home or with others outside. Overall the parents felt that respite was a good experience for the child, siblings and parents.

The Hospital Experience

The perceptions of the parents regarding the hospital service were mixed, even when parents were generally positive:

> We loved it, everyone knew us and the nurses knew how to deal with every problem. It was very old fashioned though and we kind of knew that it would have to change – Victorian institution and all that.

The main advantages of the hospital service were:

- The dormitory meant children were not alone and could be seen sooner.
- There was more and larger care and play equipment.
- There appeared to be more staff; contingencies could be dealt with more easily.
- Although the building was older, its structure and gardens were larger, enabling more flexibility in terms of single and community activity, quiet and active time.
- Because the staff comprised nurses they were able to deal with clinical incidents well within their competence. Because of this wide knowledge they also did not require repeated detailed information from parents regarding the children's care.
- During periods when parents were ill the hospital was able to provide flexible help.

However, parents also expressed disadvantages with the hospital:

- Some parents would not use the service at all, perceiving the place and service to be old fashioned and inappropriate.

- There was no follow-up or interaction with families outside the service (e.g. no liaison phone calls).
- There was little variety in terms of activity while the children were in the ward. It was a hospital model looking after patients.
- The service mainly suited immobile children with profound physical disabilities.

The New Resource Experience

Most parents were extremely pleased with the new resource. Even those parents who had liked the hospital experience described how much they valued the service and staff at the new resource. The main features of content were:

> They listen to parents.
> The children are treated like a wee family – brilliant.

These comments came from a parent who had used the hospital for many years and was extremely worried about the changes.

- Many of the staff from the hospital became staff at the new resource.
- The new resource provides a key worker who is interested with the family outside the service.
- The new resource environment is home-like, modern, light and comfortable.
- Staff are sensitive to the individual needs of the children.
- Activities for the children are much more varied than in the hospital.

> I phoned up one night at 9.45 p.m. and they were still out. That's good, I thought.

Concerns with Social Care Model: Ideology

Frustration and annoyance was expressed regarding what was seen as rigid and narrow thinking, which appeared to emanate from the social care model. The main feature of this disquiet was that communication from the new resource was sometimes patronising, with homilies about 'being good parents'.

This 'social care' model seemed to dictate that no relationship is made between chronological age and ability. This problem was seen across the services provided for their children, not just at the new resource.

One parent, to demonstrate the bizarre effect of this model, explained how her profoundly physically and mentally disabled child is taken bowling every week from school. The parent was asked to provide money for the admission and for a can of drink. The child sits in her wheelchair throughout the session, completely unable to bowl, drink from a can or partake in the personal interaction. The parent did not begrudge the money but questioned the validity of the exercise, which is carried out because, she was told, 'other children of her age go bowling'.

The social care model, which emphasises child advocacy, was perceived by some to treat parents as a barrier instead of the customer, especially as the notion of respite is as a service for the parents. Some parents resented being told that new practices, such as always accompanying their child on admission (rather than admission from school), were 'good parenting'. In effect, always having to accompany their child decreases considerably the 'respite' time in some cases. This reduces the time with other siblings, and it also brings practical difficulties:

> My only worry is that I don't drive so I would have to get a black cab – in winter [the child] would be exposed.

Despite initial apprehension and transition difficulties, there was general agreement by parents and carers that the new resource was an improvement on that at the hospital. The same is true of the approach to care and its delivery within a 'more homely' environment. There is also shared representation of the purpose of respite care in that it is for the benefit of the client, carer and family. The varied roles and activities of care staff in the new environment were acknowledged by all.

DISCUSSION FROM THE EXEMPLARS

BEARING WITNESS: PASSIVE TO ACTIVE TESTAMENT

Throughout my career as a nurse, particularly with marginalised people, the act of bearing witness has been important as a prerequisite to action. Often one cannot do something to resolve a situation immediately. The techniques described in this chapter, it is hoped, can assist the practitioner and researcher move from being a passive observer to providing active testament – something that can generate response. Another useful facet is recognising the irresolvable or main points of conflict in the present situation. This may lead toward a path of negotiated solution.

VERACITY AND RIGOUR

Qualitative research is often criticised for its lack of objectivity. However, using a rigorous design, it is possible to encapsulate truthfulness (veracity), establish context and describe 'lines of provenance'. That is, each of the stories and studies in this chapter (and others using this methodology) can be followed back to source. It is common practice to share the results and findings with the participants and respond to feedback. Of great value is that often these studies can lead to hypotheses for further, larger, quantitative, studies, giving the secondary endeavours greater accuracy and focus.

POLITICAL CHANGES: DEMOCRACY AND THE PATIENT'S PERSPECTIVE

Over recent years, particularly in the public services, there has been a move towards increased user or customer involvement. The UK National Health Service has initiated *Commissioning a Patient Led NHS* (CPLNHS). In 2006, Bill Moyes, Independent Regulator of NHS Foundation Trusts, stated how patients will not just take services that are given to them; partnership is required. Over recent years the public perception of the caring professions has been influenced by the murderous actions of a doctor, Harold Shipman, and other cases.

'We are all in charge now', one commentator has said. The need for transparency and open government has therefore increased along with personal accountability. The organised and rigorous use of collecting stories and individuals' testimony provides an effective evidence base to juxtapose competing needs and perspectives so that pathways to resolution may be achieved.

QUANTITATIVE AND QUALITATIVE: PROVIDING THE WHOLE STORY

In my own experience, the partnership between quantitative, demographic, statistical evidence and qualitative exemplars or paradigms perhaps brings us nearer to the grail of 'the whole story'. As has been seen also, of importance today in the health and social care disciplines is not just survival and overcoming death and disease. The way care is delivered and what we want have become important as well. Aspiration has to be incorporated. These facets of experience are as important in the affluent areas of the world as they are where there is deprivation – they are truly universal.

CONCLUSION

CLOSING THE CIRCLE: WILFRED OWEN'S 'PARABLE OF THE OLD MAN AND THE YOUNG'

I have always been gripped by Wilfred Owen's poetry since school days and by the work of another World War One artist, George Butterworth the composer, who died in the Battle of the Somme in 1916. About 8 years ago I travelled to Le Cateau in Picardy for the funeral of a much-loved cousin, who lived in London but wanted to be buried with her parents. St Martin's church in Le Cateau is a dark pile and was cold on the March afternoon when we buried Yolande. We proceeded to the burial at Pommereuil cemetery.

Although the name seemed familiar to me, I did not make any connection between Pommereuil and Owen (he wrote his last letter to his mother in the forester's cottage there). However, I was reading Pat Barker's *Regeneration* on my travels and as I looked over the rather flat landscape broken up by small hillocks and copses, I thought about all those men dying in their thousands for this totally unremarkable landscape. Before I went home to Glasgow I visited the Highland Regiment War Cemetery at Le Cateau and was moved to tears. Some time later I saw the film made from the book *Regeneration*, and was devastated and awestruck when the Sassoon character reads out *The Parable of the Old Man and the Young* when he hears of Owen's death. Owen's poems and photographs of the handwritten manuscripts can be viewed at www.hcu.ox.ac.uk/jtap/warpoems.htm#5.

When undertaking teaching sessions on research I often use the statistics of World War One as an example of quantitative research, asking 'What can we learn from these figures alone?'. The table I use is at www.historylearningsite.co.uk/FWWcasualties.htm. Participants usually comment on the large number of countries involved, how some countries provide very detailed numbers while others appear to be estimates and how the meaning of 'attrition' becomes more obvious.

I then read out 'Dulce et Decorum Est' about the gas attack to demonstrate the eye witness, qualitative account. Participants remark on the reality of the person who was there, how the single paradigm/vignette gives insight into the whole. I describe how in health service research we use stories and statistics in combination to tell the patient's story. We also comment on the strong political and moral message and how throughout history these personal stories come down the years.

I then read out 'Parable' and ask what information they glean from it and whether it is 'true' or not. It is such a powerful piece that it is difficult to read out loud without crying, even after several times. The discussion then turns to metaphorical truth, strong but true messages without 'facts'. I had given this lecture several times when I noticed how true the poem actually was. The last lines are:

> But the old man would not so, but slew his son, and half the seed of Europe, one by one.

Then looking at the bottom right column on the casualty statistics:

> Casualties as a percentage of total mobilised: 57%

Owen could not possibly have known this as he died before the statistics were compiled, just before the Armistice in 1918, near Le Cateau on the Ors-Sambre Canal. The three pieces thus form a circle, a whole truth. Listening to George Butterworth's 'Banks of Green Willow' augments this truth as one reflects how shameful is the destruction of all that is beautiful.

I hope this chapter has created some paradigm shifts for the reader and also provided a fitting end to the contributions of my colleagues in this book.

REFERENCES

Atkinson, J. (1993) When somebody knows my name – report on a care project for care of 200 HIV positive children in Romania. Radix Journal October, p. 7.

Atkinson, J. (2000) *Nursing Homeless Men: A Study of Proactive Intervention*. John Wiley & Sons, Chichester.

Atkinson, J., Kennedy, E. (2002) *Who are you to tell me what good parenting is?* Findings from a descriptive study of stakeholders at a respite centre for severely disabled children in South-West Scotland. Full paper published in Proceedings, Nursing Research Conference, Trinity College Dublin, November 2002.

Atkinson, J., Kennedy, E., Goldsworthy, S., Drummond, S. (2002) Patients' cancer journeys in Kintyre – a qualitative study of the care, support and information needs of people with cancer and their careers. *European Journal of Oncology Nursing* **6**(2), 85–92.

Benner, P. (1984) *From Novice to Expert: Excellence and Power in Clinical Nursing Practice*. Addison-Wesley, Menlo Park, CA.

Burnard, P. (1991) *Counselling Skills for Health Professionals*. Chapman & Hall, London.

Callan, L., Gilbert, T., Golding, K., Lockyer, T., Rafter, K. (1995) Assessing health needs in people with severe learning disabilities: a qualitative approach. *Journal of Clinical Nursing* **4**, 295–302.

Carr, E. (1999) Talking on the telephone with people who have experienced pain in hospital: clinical audit or research? *Journal of Advanced Nursing* **29**(1), 194–200.

Fennell, D. (1988) *Investigation into the King's Cross Underground Fire*. The Stationery Office Books, London.

Flanagan, J. C. (1954) The critical incident technique. *Psychological Bulletin* **51**(4), 327–358.

Hall, S. (1996) An exploration of parental perception of the nature and level of support needed to care for their child with special needs. *Journal of Advanced Nursing* **24**, 512–521.

Kirk, S. (1998) Trends in community care and patient participation: implications for the roles of informal carers and community nurses in the United Kingdom. *Journal of Advanced Nursing* **28**, 370–381.

McPherson, K., Leydon, G. (Principal Investigators) (2001) The information and support needs of cancer patients. Research study funded by the Cancer Research Campaign (March 1998–May 2001), London School of Hygiene and Tropical Medicine.

Nolan, M., Grant, G., Keady, J. (1996) *Understanding Family Care. A Multi-Dimensional Model of Caring and Coping*. Open University Press, Milton Keynes.

Norman, I., Parker, F. (1990) Psychiatric patients' views of their lives before and after moving to a hostel: a qualitative study. *Journal of Advanced Nursing* **15**, 1036–1044.

Norman, I. J., Redfern, S. J., Tomalin, D. A., Oliver, S. (1992) Developing Flanagan's critical incident technique to elicit indicators of high and low quality nursing care from patients and their nurses. *Journal of Advanced Nursing* **17**, 590–600.

O'Mahony, M. (2001) Women's lived experience of breast biopsy: a phenomenological study. *Journal of Clinical Nursing* **10**(4), 512–520.

Patton, M. Q. (1990) *Qualitative Evaluation and Research Methods*. Sage, Newbury Park, CA.

Schwartz, A. (2003) Researching the human spirit. *UCSF Magazine* **23**(2). Available at: pub.ucsf.edu/magazine/200306/spirit.html. Accessed April 2006.

Strauss, A. L., Corbin, J. (1998) *Basics of Qualitative Research: Techniques and Procedures for Developing Grounded Theory*, 2nd edn. Sage, Newbury Park, CA.

Vanleit, B., Crowe, T. K. (2000) Promoting well-being in mothers of children with disabilities. *OT Practice* **5**(13), 26–31.

Worth, A., McIntosh, J., Carney, O., Lugton, J. (1995) Assessment of need for district nursing. Department of Nursing and Community Health, Glasgow Caledonian University.

Zigmond, A. S., Snaith, R. P. (1983) The Hospital Anxiety and Depression Scale. *Acta Psychiatrica Scandinavica* **67**, 361–370.

Index

Note: 'n.' after a page reference indicates there is a note on that page.